PAIN-FREE
ARTHRITIS

PAIN-FREE ARTHRITIS

by Dvera Berson with Sander Roy

S & J BOOKS

Published by S & J Books
387 Ocean Parkway
Brooklyn, New York 11218

Drawings by David Dowland and Joyce Smith

Photographs reproduced by kind permission of Joyce Milberg

ISBN: 0-9609608-0-5

Library of Congress Catalogue Card Number 82-61677

Earlier Edition published in Great Britain by New English Library

CONTENTS

THIS BOOK IS DEDICATED TO MILTON AND JOYCE
WITHOUT WHOM MY LIFE AND THIS BOOK WOULDN'T
HAVE BEEN POSSIBLE

Preface

This is the true story of how I used *pain-free* special water exercises to conquer crippling arthritis. It tells how I used them to *gradually relax, stretch* and *strengthen* the muscles surrounding my joints and thus gradually eliminate all feelings of pain and stiffness from my body.

When I was sixty years old, I had been suffering from arthritis for six years and I was getting progressively worse. I wore a neck-brace and a back-support, slept in a hospital bed, did traction three times a day, had deformed fingers, and was in constant pain. My condition was diagnosed as being rheumatoid arthritis and osteoarthritis, osteoporisis and cervical spondylosis deformans. The ways things were going, I was in very real danger of becoming permanently crippled, but I didn't stand by and let this happen to me. I did something about it.

Today, at age sixty-five, my pains are one hundred per cent better and my fingers are no longer deformed. I sleep in a regular bed and no longer need back or neck support. I have progressed from being unable to sign my name without severe pain to being able to swim the backstroke 100-150 lengths of a pool, totalling up to a mile and a half.

I have medical records, doctor's bills, X-rays, blood tests, drug bills, and hospital records to document what my condition was. I tell you this because people meeting me today for the first time would never know that I had ever suffered from serious arthritis.

Today, the only limitations with my condition are that I can't lift heavy objects without some pain and that if I stop water exercising for two weeks I start to feel some pain and stiffness return to my hands and neck. Otherwise, when I keep up with my water exercises I can carry on all normal activities without any pain whatsoever.

What I accomplished was the result of a special programme that I developed myself.

The Arthritis Foundation and most reputable arthritis

doctors recommend proper exercise as being very beneficial in the treatment of arthritis. The problem with exercises that doctors recommend is that they are too painful to do for someone already in pain. I personally experienced this problem. In the first years of my illness, my specialist sent me to a physiotherapist for arthritis exercises. The exercises that he gave me hurt me so severely that I was forced to discontinue them. The reason that I was able to persevere with my special water exercises is that they are absolutely pain free.

What they accomplished was to gradually relax, stretch and strenghten the muscles surrounding my joints. Over a period of weeks and months of relaxing, stretching and strengthening, my body became progressively less painful and more flexible. Eventually, all feelings of pain and stiffness were eliminated from my body.

Starting ten minutes a day with pain-free special water exercises, I changed my life. If you, or someone you care for, suffers from arthritis, you owe it to yourself to read this book.

Most people have come to accept their arthritis pain the way they accept death and taxes. They are very unhappy about the situation but feel there is little or nothing they can do about it. This book was written to announce that now there is something they can do about it, if they really want to.

The arthritis pain-relief programme described in this book does not involve changing your diet slightly, nor does it involve swallowing a new miracle drug. What it does involve is your expending effort to help yourself. The disadvantage of my special water exercise programme is that it isn't an instant magic cure. The advantage is that it really works! That is the most important thing about this book. It offers people who want to help themselves the knowledge of how to really do it.

It is not my intention, though, to suggest this programme is a replacement for a patient's doctor. Hopefully, this programme will be of help to both doctor and patient in treating the patient's arthritis pain. The self-help aspect of this book comes into being because doctors do not have pools in their offices and they don't have the time to go to pools to

supervise and encourage the individual exercise programmes of every one of their patients.

General exercise principles are repeated on a separate page
in special type every now and then throughout the twenty-
five beginner's-exercise descriptions. I risked boring you
with such repetition only because of the importance to you
of understanding why these principles have to be empha-
sised. If you do not pay strict attention to them, the rest of the
programme will be rendered ineffective.

The books I have read about arthritis fall into two
categories: quack books that offer simple, easy solutions that
don't work, and legitimate general-information books that
tell you everything about arthritis except what you should
do about it. This book is a legitimate attempt to help you
help yourself. I tried to treat you not as a nameless patient
but rather as a sensitive human being who happens to be in a
lot of pain. I tell you about my own suffering and recovery to
inspire you to achieve your own recovery. This book does
not attempt to be a general-information book about
arthritis. I have tried to include only information that would
be of direct benefit to you in improving your condition.

DVERA BERSON

Part One

1 My Life Before

What follows is a brief history of what I suffered physically and mentally before my life changed for the better.

I didn't think it could happen to me, except that it did. I always thought arthritis was something that happend to 'old people'. When this all started I was fifty-four and I didn't consider myself old. I didn't know what arthritis was doing bothering me. In fact, at first I didn't even know I had arthritis.

It started with a pain in my jawbone, for which I naturally went to a dentist. I felt relieved when my dentist couldn't find anything wrong with my teeth or gums.

The pain persisted and so did I. I went to my internist, who gave me Indocid for my jaw. After a few weeks the pain went away and I thought no more about it.

Six months later, seemingly out of nowhere I developed excruciating pains in my neck, back, hands and the lower back of my head. This all happened over one terrible weekend. My internist told me I had arthritis. He put me on a programme of taking eight Bufferins a day.

On one of my subsequent visits, when I complained about the pain, my doctor told me, 'You have to learn to live with it.' That statement convinced me to change doctors. Even at that stage, when my pains were a lot less than they were to become, there was no way I could learn to live with them.

I decided to get expert advice, so I called the Arthritis Foundation. They recommended an arthritis clinic not far from where I lived. At the clinic, they took X-rays and blood tests, both of which confirmed that I had rheumatoid arthritis, osteoporosis and osteoarthritis. I went to this clinic for about three months. The doctors there prescribed medication for me which did not help at all.

After this, on the recommendation of a friend of mine, I went to an internist who made every effort to help me

—first with cortisone and then with two series of gold treatments. When I was taking these treatments my pains stopped getting worse and were, in fact, about twenty-five per cent better. The unfortunate thing about both cortisone and gold is that, because of harmful side effects (see page 102), you can take only a limited number of shots before being forced to discontinue the treatment.

After five and a half years of various treatments, my neck got so bad that it was decided to put me in the hospital for supervised traction. I had twenty-one days of private health coverage, so that was my allotted time for recovery. As it was, I had only three days of traction. It turned out that I was lucky this happened, because the traction I received for three days was the opposite of the kind I needed.

I found this out by going to an orthopaedic surgeon affiliated to a different hospital. After a thorough examination he, at least, prescribed a way to give me outpatient traction that helped rather than hurt my condition. After a few months of correct traction my neck improved to the point where the pain was awful but bearable. The pain was especially bearable since the surgeon had told me that the only alternative to enduring it was having an operation on my neck.

Over a six-year period, because of cortisone and gold treatments and probably because of the natural course of the disease, my condition didn't decline in a straight line. I had 'good' periods as well as 'bad' periods. The problem with my 'good' periods was that they seemed good only when compared to my 'bad' periods. I was always in pain. Also in each succeeding 'good' period my condition was worse than it had been in the previous 'good' period.

My condition declined down a series of plateaux rather than in a straight line, but over a period of time the decline was nevertheless relentless. After six years of spending countless money and effort to help myself, I had 'improved' to the point where I was wearing a neck-brace and a back-support and doing over-the-door traction three times a day. My hands were crippled and I was in constant pain.

MY MENTAL AND EMOTIONAL CONDITION

I wish I could say that during my trials and tribulations with doctors and hospitals I always kept my head high and my spirit strong. But it was not like that. First of all, I couldn't keep my head high. Physically, my condition was such that I had to walk with a stoop. Unfortunately, my mental and emotional condition matched my physical condition.

Aside from the pain, the hardest thing to live with was not having any hope of recovery. I am a fairly strong person, and I think I could have endured anything if I had known that at some point my suffering would end and I would survive. After a while it looked as if the only time my pains were going to stop was when I stopped existing.

When my first internist told me, 'You have to learn to live with it', my first reaction was one of defiance. I said to myself, 'What does he know? I'll find a doctor who can help me.' Three years later my reaction was quite different when I showed a doctor in whom I had more confidence the three fingers on my right hand that were gnarled and deformed and giving me excruciating pain. I asked, 'Doctor, do I have to wait to undergo this torture with every finger?' He replied, 'That's a very difficult question to answer.' That answer depressed me as much as the pain.

There I was, going to the best internist I could find, doing everything he said, and on a year-to-year basis I was worse every year. It got to the point where I would lie in my darkened bedroom and just cry to myself without tears, 'Why me?' My condition was so bad that I wasn't ever physically comfortable. I used a cervical pillow when lying in bed, but even that didn't help. I couldn't lie for more than ten minutes at a time without having to change my position.

I had the same problem trying to sit for more than ten minutes at a time. There was a two-hour waiting time at my doctor's office. I had to spend the two hours alternating between sitting for ten minutes and standing for ten minutes with my back leaning against the wall for support.

Before all this happened to me, I was a divorcée with hopes of remarriage but with no one special in mind.

Afterwards, one of the things I would think about in my darkened room was, 'Who would want me now?' While I still hoped to be married to someone I could care for, that marriage could take place only in a world now hopelessly lost to me — a world where my pains and deformity didn't exist. The way things really were, I had no interest in any people, male or female. As I retreated into myself, everyone else's problems and concerns seemed very petty to me. The only reality was me and my pain.

While I am admitting other unpleasant thoughts that I had at the time, let me admit that I was also ashamed of myself. I wasn't ashamed of feeling sorry for myself or being involved with myself to the exclusion of everything else. Rather, I was ashamed of being a cripple.

In the winter I could hide my hands with gloves. I always wore my back-support under my clothes. What I couldn't stand was having to wear my cervical collar in public. I told casual acquaintances that my collar was for a pinched nerve. I told strangers who met me for the first time that I was suffering from whiplash.

Generally I was frustrated, unhappy and practically hopeless. In my darkened room, I began to think that my life was over.

Looking back on those six years of suffering, I think this state of depression helped contribute to the worsening of my condition. It was a vicious circle. Being tense, nervous, and unhappy caused my muscles to become tenser and tighter, which in turn caused more pain. This in turn caused me to be even more tense and nervous. At the time, I was dimly aware of the situation, but there was nothing I could do about it.

As long as I was in constant pain and without real hope, I found it impossible to be happy or positive. Once I started doing water exercises and felt a tangible physical improvement, I found it a lot easier to be cheerful and to begin, once more, to enjoy life.

2 My Exercise History

In the six years that I spent waiting for someone else to help me, I was treated by two specialists and two physiotherapists, consulted with an orthopaedic surgeon, was hospitalised for traction, used a hydrocollator for my neck and paraffin for my hands and also received cortisone injections and two series of gold injections, plus countless oral medication. None of these treatments proved to have any lasting benefit.

The only treatment that has ever provided me with complete and lasting relief is the muscle-relaxing water exercise programme which I developed.

Now, as I write, I have absolutely no pain. I can proudly walk with my head up. I don't wear a cervical collar or use a back-support or do any traction. I don't take drugs or visit doctors for arthritis. My fingers are no longer deformed.

The principle of exercising in water is a simple one. Movement is much easier in water than out of it. On dry land every movement is a fight against gravity. In the water, you are lighter and more mobile, because your body is being supported by the buoyancy of the water. Exercises that cause pain and strain when done on dry land can become easy and pain free when done in the water.

I started my exercises at an outdoor pool, while I was on a three-month holiday in Florida. I have to admit that at the the time I didn't have any grand design for curing myself. I had two main thoughts when I started. One was the hope of doing a little something to improve my condition. The other was the fear of doing something to hurt myself badly.

When I started I was amazed at the freedom from pain I had when I moved. Even so, I confined myself to slow gentle movement and made sure to rest as soon as I felt the least bit tired. I exercised every day, and by the end of the first week I noticed some slight improvement. During the next three months I increased my stamina and flexibility by gradually lengthening the time I spent on each exercise and gradually increasing my radius of movement. What happened was that I was slowly loosening and relaxing my muscles, while at the same time strengthening them.

The obvious improvement in my physical condition, and the knowledge that it was because of something I myself was doing, gave me a tremendous psychological lift. Having hope for the first time in years definitely helped relax my mind. As I became more relaxed and less tense mentally, my muscles relaxed even more. I am sure that the interreacton of mental, physical and emotional improvement helped speed my recovery.

By the end of the three months in Florida, while I wasn't yet well, I was considerably better. My pains were much less severe. I had more general stamina and I had a much greater interest in doing things other than worrying about myself.

Unaccountably, when I returned to New York I didn't immediately continue with my water exercises. I can't remember exactly why. Possibly I thought I was permanently better. Possibly, I wasn't yet a hundred per cent convinced that my exercises were the sole things responsible for my improvement. And possibly, after feeling better, I became lazy. In Florida, I could walk out of my hotel room and into the pool thirty seconds later. In New York, it's a lot more trouble to find and travel to a pool.

After being back in New York six weeks and seeing slow changes for the worse in my conditon, I remembered how much better I felt in Florida and made up my mind to join a health club. After two weeks there, my condition improved to the level it had been in Florida. It kept right on improving, and after a while I felt confident enough to start doing the backstroke. For my condition, this was the perfect exercise. In a relaxed position on my back I can exercise my wrists, arms, shoulders, neck, back, hips, and feet all in one motion. Even today, when I have no pain, I swim slowly and in a relaxed manner and pause at one end of the pool. My current regimen consists of forty-five minutes of doing the backstroke and one other advanced exercise, three minutes in the whirlpool, and then forty-five minutes of the same exercises, finishing with three minutes in the sauna.

Even though I have made tremendous progress in my condition, eliminating pain, swelling and deformity from my body, I am not cured. Recently I was on holiday in California, visiting relatives. I was relaxed mentally. Physically I encountered no strain and enjoyed myself immensely, visiting, sight-seeing and eating out. Yet at the end of a pleasant month of not exercising in California, I felt stiffer and tighter throughout my body. I also had slight pains in my neck and hands.

Back in New York, after a week of exercising, my condition came back to normal. This further proved to me that I'm not cured, but rather involved in a lifetime discipline of helping myself.

3 How the Exercises Work

As I've pointed out, this exercise programme, even if done properly, will not cure you of arthritis. What it will do is effectively treat the symptoms of arthritis so that you can eliminate your pain and regain flexibility. Arthritis is a disease of the joints, but it is in the muscles surrounding the joints that you feel most of your arthritis pain and stiffness. Tense, tight muscles press on nerve endings. Weak and tense muscles make movement painful and difficult.

My special water exercise programme treats your pain by treating your muscles. It gradually *relaxes, stretches* and *strengthens* tense, tight and weak muscles. Over a period of time as your muscles gradually relax, stretch and strengthen, your joints become progressively less painful and more flexible.

Since these exercises are virtually pain free, you don't have to worry about torturing yourself in the hope of seeing improvement. But you do have to have patience. You can't expect to exercise for one day, or one week, and see great improvement. These exercises will work for you, but they are not magic. After a few weeks you can expect slight improvement, and after a few months you can expect major improvement.

By doing these exercises regularly, you gradually increase the strength and flexibility of your muscles. If you don't do them regularly, all the benefit is lost. Every time you exercise, there is a slight, unnoticeable increase in muscle strength. Imagine your muscle strength as being 100 units of strength. After exercising one day, you build yourself up to 101 units of strength. If you exercise the next day, you start at 101 units and build yourself up to 102 units. If instead of exercising the next day you wait a few days, you would have to start all over again at 100 units of strength.

By exercising every day or at least five times a week, you build your strength and flexibility progressively. On a day-to-day basis, this increase will not be noticeable but on a month-to-month basis your progress will be amazing.

Once you have achieved the desired results of eliminating your pain and increasing your flexibility, you can congratulate yourself. But you cannot retire from your exercise programme. Remember, you have not cured yourself of arthritis. You have merely controlled the symptoms.

If you stop doing your water exercises, you will find your units of stength decreasing just as steadily as they increased before. Gradually, you will again become aware of discomfort and impaired movement. To prevent this from happening, you must continue doing your exercises three times a week as a maintenance programme for the rest of your life.

Once you have seen the benefits of these exercises, and how enjoyable they are to do, you won't resent that fact. Instead you will love this regimen as much as I do.

A LITTLE INSPIRATION

It is very simple. If you want to help yourself you can. You don't have to endure pain and physical suffering. You don't have to endure the mental anguish of wondering how much worse you are going to get. You can look forward to a life free of pain and deformity. All you have to do is be willing to make a continuous effort to help yourself.

With my special water exercises you don't have to endure additional pain. You don't have to worry about hurting yourself. You can concentrate on helping yourself.

For the purpose of doing exercises beneficial to your arthritis condition, think of the water as the best friend you have. Any time you move any part of your body in the water, that movement is much easier and much less painful than the same movement on dry land. The buoyancy of the water makes your body feel almost weightless. Every movement is less of a strain. Exercises that are too painful to do on dry land can become pleasant to do when done in the water.

Don't take my word for it. Go to a pool and see for yourself. Without signing up for a long-term membership, ask to try the facilities, or pay for one day. Being careful to follow instructions, try the beginner's exercises illustrated in the next chapter that pertain to your condition. See for yourself how much easier they are to do in the water than out of it. Then prepare to dedicate yourself to helping yourself.

If you are willing to follow instructions and put in the required effort, you can change your life.

CONFIRMATION

Before you start reading the exercise section of this book I want to emphasise an important point. What I say about arthritis pain being caused by tense, tight and weak muscles is not just my pet theory to explain my recovery. That arthritis pain is felt in the muscles and caused by tense, tight muscles pressing on nerve ends is a medically accepted fact. It is also a medically accepted fact that weak and tense muscles make movement painful and difficult.

The popular misconception that arthritis pain is caused by deterioration of the bones is exactly that, a popular misconception. Deterioration of the bones and joints is certainly involved in arthritis but is only occasionally the direct cause of arthritis pain. Tense, tight and weak muscles are the direct cause of almost all arthritis pain. Once you accept that fact you can easily accept the thesis that effectively treating your muscles will reduce and eliminate your arthritis pain.

The special water exercise programme you will read about in the next chapters does effectively treat your muscles. By adhering to this programme I dramatically changed my life for the better. You can do the the same.

CHRONIC BACK AND NECK PAIN

This special water exercise programme should be very beneficial to many people who suffer from chronic back and neck pain not involving arthritis. First check with your doctor to determine the cause of your pain. Then ask your doctor if effectively treating your muscles and ligaments would reduce your pain. There is a strong likelihood that it would.

While tense, tight and weak muscles are not responsible for everything bad in this world, they do play a major part in causing most chronic back and neck pain. Simply put, the problem is that your muscles are not strong enough to properly support your skeletal system. Conservative treatment suggests wearing cumbersome surgical corsets and cervical collars to provide added support for your back and neck. My programme suggests gradual strengthening of your muscles so that they can perform their natural function without the need for collars and corsets.

I have two reasons for mentioning chronic back and neck pain in a book supposedly devoted exclusively to arthritis. The first is their similar common cause of pain. The second is my wish that people suffering from chronic back and neck pain should achieve a similar happy result from their treatment.

General Information about the Exercises and Exercise Facilities

1. If your problem is arthritis of the fingers, wrists, toes or ankles, you can derive benefits from doing my water exercises at home in your bathtub. Arthritis of the elbows, shoulders, neck, back, hips and knees requires a larger body of water to work in. Climate permitting, these exercises can be done in an outdoor pool or the sea. To exercise the year round in a city, as in my case, you have to find access to a pool.

2. Using an indoor pool doesn't have to be an expensive proposition. In addition to public swimming-baths, health clubs, organisations like YMCAs, YWCAs, schools and many other organisations have pools. The health club where I belong gives a fifty per cent discount to people over sixty-two and does not ask proof of age. Before signing any contracts try the various facilities at least once and inquire about discounts. Do not let yourself be pressured to your disadvantage by aggressive salesmen. Also there, is a possibility that if your doctor prescribes this programme for you, the Inland Revenue could allow the costs as a medical deduction you can take on your income tax.

3. It is very inconvenient to have to go to a pool five times a week, but that inconvenience is nothing when compared to the good it does. I travel back and forth by bus, and I don't enjoy waiting for buses, especially in the winter. I find, though, that whatever inconvenience and discomfort this brings is a thousand times better than being in pain. The same rationale applies to the expense involved in joining and travelling to a health club, and by spending money to join a pool, I'm saving on prescriptions.

4. The water in the pool doesn't have to be any particular temperature, as along as it doesn't feel chilly. Also the air temperature in the area around the pool shouldn't be colder than the water. Even today, with my condition a hundred per cent better, I never swim in cold water or take cold showers.

5. When I started doing my water exercises, I did the exercises every day, weather permitting. This was because I was very enthusiastic about them, and because travelling to the pool was no problem. If travelling or other commitments make everyday exercise inconvenient to you, five times a week is the acceptable minimum to start with. Once you have achieved your desired goals, a maintenance programme of three times a week is sufficient to prevent relapse. If it is a physical impossibility for you to get to a pool five times a week, you are better off going three times a week than not going at all. If you start three or four times a week you will definitely improve. The only drawback is that your improvement won't be fast, and it may or may not be as complete.

6. When I say that these exercises are pain free I mean that they do not cause any additional pain. That doesn't mean that your pains will miraculously disappear as soon as you enter the water. What it means is that properly exercising in the water causes no more pain than being motionless on dry land.

Exercise that does cause increased pain not only is uncomfortable but also is bad for you. Increased pain causes increased muscle tightness, which in turn causes even more pain. Exercise without increased pain is good for you because it causes muscles to relax and stretch, and thus reduces your pain. That is why exercise that causes increased pain should be avoided, and exercise that doesn't should be encouraged.

The water makes exercise much easier to do. Exercising in the water should not cause additional pain. If you do experience some additional pain it is because you are trying to do too much too soon. Lessen your exercise repetitions and/or range of motion. Find a level of exercise that is comfortable for you and then gradually build yourself up from there. If you do things moderately, you shouldn't experience any additional pain.

7. All my movements in the water are of a slow and gentle nature. The idea is to *relax, stretch* and *strengthen* the muscles, not strain them.

8. To exercise for an hour requires much more muscle strength than to exercise for five minutes. That is why you should always strive to increase the amount of time you spend exercising. You'll know you are doing enough in the water when you reach the point where, on dry land, you are no longer in pain. When I started, I did each exercise for about a minute. My general rule was that when I was tired or felt any slight strain, I stopped and rested. In time, as I became more flexible and increased my general stamina, I was able to exercise for longer periods of time without feeling any additional strain. Increases in duration of exercise time didn't follow any preconceived plan. They followed naturally from the improvement of my condition.

9. When I started I didn't have the full range of movement to do most of the exercises completely. I didn't worry about it. I started doing them partially, and gradually built up my flexibility. Let me emphasise again that slow and gentle movements in the water lead to steady, gradual improvements in stamina, muscle strength and flexibility.

10. Nowhere in this book do I ever tell you to do an exercise for five minutes or to repeat it ten times. Each person's condition is different from everyone else's. The fact that I could do an exercise ten times when I began exercising has nothing to do with you. You might be able to do it thirty times, or only one time and then only partially. When you are exercising it is important that you do only as much as is comfortable for you to do and then try to improve from there. Improvement doesn't depend on how much you can do in the beginning. It depends on how much you persevere.

11. I make it a rule always to go to the pool at off hours, when it is least crowded. When I swim or do my other exercises, I'm very careful of other people. I don't want to injure anyone or be injured myself. Occasionally I find inconsiderate people who swim as if they are the only ones in the pool. I make it my business to watch out for them. I also pick out fixed points in the ceiling under which I will swim. That enables me to keep my course straight.

12. After I've finished my exercises, showered and dressed, I rest at least twenty minutes before going home. I do this especially in the winter, to make sure that the cold outside-air isn't a shock after the warmth of the pool.

13. It is important to emphasise that you do not need the expensive facilities of a health club. The health club where I belong has a beautiful well-equipped gymnasium. I manage to avoid it like the plague. To this day, I will not exercise on dry land. Why should I? If I try to demonstrate the twisting motion of the backstroke even once on dry land, I feel a slight strain. In the water, I can swim the backstroke for an hour wihtout feeling any strain whatsoever.

14. Most health club pools have a whirlpool. This is nice —but again is not essential. At the halfway point in my exercises, I go into the whirlpool for three minutes. I sit with the water up to my chin. I also make sure to sit between the jets so that the force of the jets doesn't hurt me. The whirlpool isn't necessary for my exercise programme, but it gives a pleasant and relaxing sensation. After the whirlpool, I slowly re-enter the pool and submerge myself up to my neck to readjust my body temperature. When I start to swim again, I start especially slowly so as to gradually get myself back into the rhythm of things.

15. A word of caution about the use of both the sauna and the whirlpool: stay no longer than three minutes in either one. On more than one occasion I have seen someone go into the whirlpool for the first time, spend fifteen minutes there, and then have to be carried out. By the way, from the arthritis standpoint, there is no reason for spending too much time in either the sauna or the whirlpool. Heat treatments of any sort temporarily relax your muscles but provide no permanent benefit.

16. If I have been on holiday or have had a virus or for some other reason have been unable to do my water exercises, for a week or two I do only eighty or ninety per cent as much as I did the last time. Each occasion is different, but usually after a few sessions I'm able to work myself back comfortably to where I was.

17. This book outlines a self-help programme that will help you greatly, but self-help does not mean self-diagnosis. Before starting this programme I suggest you check with your doctor. If it hasn't already been done, your doctor can determine if you actually have arthritis. Just because you have pains that seem like arthritis it doesn't necessarily mean than you have arthritis. Your doctor can also determine if you have some physical condition other than arthritis that might be adversely affected by this form of moderate exercise.

Here is a word of obvious medical caution. In one of the early stages of rheumatoid arthritis, some people develop a fever. If you have such a fever you should not attempt pool exercise. You should, however, discuss my special water exercise programme with your doctor. He will tell you how soon after the fever subsides you can start an exercise programme.

18. All exercise movement should feel as if you are *pushing* and/or *lifting* the water. When you get this feeling it means that you are using the water to provide slight resistance to your movement. This resistance helps to increase your muscle strength.

19. The exercises are divided into beginner's, intermediate and advanced exercises. Start with the beginner's exercises appropriate to your condition. Some beginner's exercises should be replaced by intermediate and advanced exercises as soon as you are able to do so. Others do not have an effective intermediate or advanced replacement, so they must be continued. The procedure you should follow is noted under each beginner's exercise.

20. Don't worry about not being able to do the beginner's exercises. Before I started my exercise programme, I hadn't exercised in over forty years. These exercises were specially written for people who never exercise, and who additionally are in a great deal of pain.

21. Make sure you try to do all the beginner's exercises that apply to your condition, not just the ones you like best. These exercises are designed to be used in combination with one another, so as to put your muscles through their full range of motion and thus provide the maximum benefit for you.

4 Your First Day of Exercise

Do not attempt to do too much. Your first day should be a testing process to determine what you can and cannot comfortably do. Try the various exercises that apply to your particular condition. Even if you find all the exercises easy, do not overdo any of them. If you do overdo an exercise, you might not feel badly in the pool but could experience increased discomfort within the following twenty-four hours. If this happens do not be discouraged, just wait a few days and then do much less the next time you exercise. Remember, your muscles are not used to exercise and they must be gradually built up.

If you experience increased discomfort from trying to duplicate the full range of motion pictured in a drawing, then only do the exercise partly. Make sure that you do all your exercise repetitions within a range of motion that is comfortable for you. In ensuing days and weeks try to gradually increase both your range of motion and the number of repetitions you do. Do not be discouraged if the drawing shows a thirty-six-inch range of motion and you can only move three inches comfortably. Keep trying and you will experience gradual progressive improvement.

When you are doing three or four exercises for a particular condition it is possible that one of them may be too uncomfortable for you to do even partly. If that is the case then don't force yourself to do it. Do the other exercises for a month and then try the hard one again. If you still can't do it, then try again a month later. Eventually the other exercises will build you up to the point where you will indeed be able to do the one or the ones that gave you difficulty.

It is much easier to exercise in water than on land. The probability is that if you are careful you will not experience any increased discomfort. If you do experience some discomfort the first day it is because you exceeded the limits of what is comfortable for you to do. Sometimes that is unavoidable because you can't know your limits until you test them. The important thing, though, is to find a level of exercise that is comfortable for you. Once you do that, the battle is almost won. The rest is just a matter of gradual increase in range of motion and number of repetitions. Remember, don't overdo anything the first days or weeks. If you are content to start slowly and improve gradually, you will be very satisfied with your final result.

The Exercise
Programme

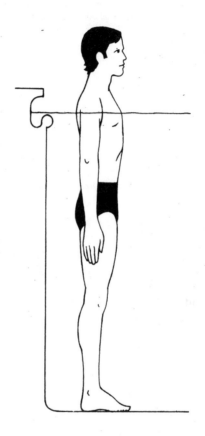

WHERE AND HOW TO STAND

When doing exercises for your arms, stand with your back near the edge of the pool so that you don't have to worry about careless swimmers colliding with your back. When doing these exercises, make sure the water is always above the part being exercised. If you are doing ankle exercises, but additionally have a problem with low-back pains, stand in water well above the area of pain so that you get maximum support for that sector while exercising your ankle.

5 Beginner's Exercises

The following instructions apply to each and every one of the twenty-five beginner's exercises.

Do an exercise for as long as you comfortably can without its becoming a strain. When you become tired, it is important that you stop and rest. After resting, repeat the exercise if you can.

In the beginning, if you can't even do any or all of these exercises for very long, or if you don't have the full range of movement pictured, it is important to have patience with yourself. In time your stamina and flexibility will increase naturally, and it will become much easier to do each exercise for longer periods of time with a greater radius of movement. The rule is always to try to do a little more than you did the last time, if you can do it without increasing the strain on yourself.

There is almost no benefit from doing these exercises once or twice a week. They should be done at least five times a week at the beginning. Then, once you have achieved your desired results, you can reduce to a three-times-a-week maintenance programme. Remember, results take time.

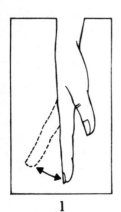
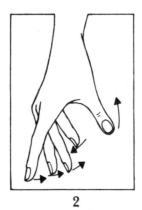
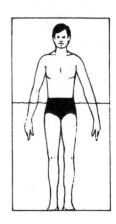

1   2

Exercise 1 — To *relax, stretch* and *strengthen* the muscles surrounding your finger joints.

Stand in water to your waist with your hands comfortably at your sides as shown. Then flutter your fingers. Move each of your fingers forward and backard the way the one finger in Figure 1 is being moved. All your fingers should be moving at the same time, but they should be moving independently. As some fingers are moving forward others should be moving backward as shown in Figure 2. Notice that the thumb movement is up and down, not backward and forward. If you find this thumb movement awkward, don't worry about it. In time your thumb will more easily co-ordinate with the rest of your fingers. All finger movement should feel as if you are *pushing* the water. All movement should be *slow* and *gentle*.

This exercise quite possibly can be done at home in a bathtub or basin, but take note of the caution spelled out on page 80.

The exercise should be continued regardless of the advanced exercises you do.

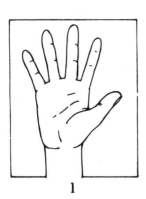 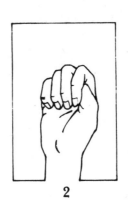 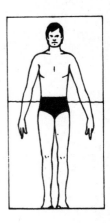

1   2

Exercise 2 — Further to *relax, stretch* and *strengthen* the muscles surrounding your finger joints.

Stand in water to your waist with your hands comfortably at your sides as shown. With your palms facing towards your body, open each hand and stretch your fingers as much as you comfortably can, as shown in Figure 1. Then attempt to clench your fist as shown in Figure 2. All opening and closing motions should feel as if you are *pushing* the water forward and backward. All movement should be *slow* and *gentle*.

If you intend to do the exercise at home, see the caution on page 80.

This exercise should be continued regardless of the advanced exercises you do.

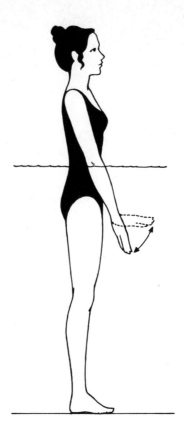

Exercise 3 — To *relax, stretch* and *strengthen* the muscles surrounding your wrist joints.

Stand in water to your waist. Without raising your arm, raise your hand below the wrist as high as you can and then lower it as far as you can. All raising and lowering motions should feel as if you are *pushing* and *lifting* the water. All movements should be *slow* and *gentle*.

If you intend to do the exercise at home, see the caution on page 80.

This exercise should be replaced with Exercises 32 and 33 as soon as you are able to do so.

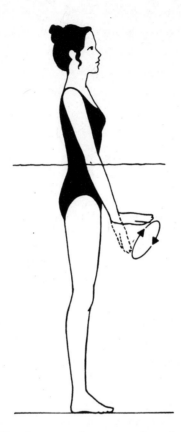

Exercise 4 — Further to *relax, stretch* and *strengthen* the muscles surrounding your wrist joints.

Stand in water to your waist. Rotate your hand below the wrist so that you feel as if you are *pushing* the water around in a circular motion. Rotation should be to the right for a period of time and then to the left for a period of time. All movement should take place in your hand below the wrist. Try not to move your upper arm. All movement should be *slow* and *gentle*.

If you intend to do the exercise at home, see the caution on page 80.

This exercise should be continued regardless of the advanced exercises you do.

Do these exercises for as long as you comfortably can without their becoming a strain. When you become tired, it is important that you stop and rest. After resting, repeat the exercise if you can.

In the beginning, if you can't even do any or all of these exercises for very long, or if you don't have the full range of movement pictured, it is important to have patience with yourself. In time your stamina and flexibility will increase naturally, and it will become much easier to do each exercise for longer periods of time with a greater radius of movement. The rule is always to try to do a little more than you did the last time, if you can do it without increasing the strain on yourself.

There is almost no benefit from doing these exercises once or twice a week. They should be done at least five times a week at the beginning. Then, once you have achieved your desired results, you can reduce to a three-times-a-week maintenance programme. Remember, results take time.

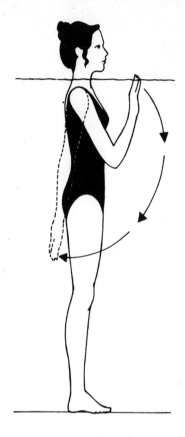

Exercise 5 — To *relax, stretch* and *strengthen* the muscles surrounding your elbow joints.

Stand in water above your shoulders. Raise and lower your arm below the elbow so that on the raising and lowering motions you feel as if you are *lifting* the water up and *pushing* the water down. All movement should be *slow* and *gentle*.

This exercise should be replaced with Exercises 32 and 33 as soon as you are able to do so.

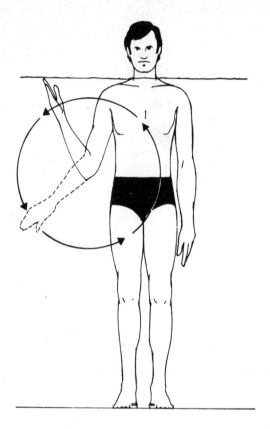

Exercise 6 — Further to *relax, stretch* and *strengthen* the muscles surrounding your elbow joints.

Stand in water above your shoulders. Rotate your arms below the elbow so that you feel as if you are *pushing* the water around in a circular motion. (To complete the circle you will have to adjust the position of your elbow.) Rotation should be to the right for a period of time and then to the left for a period of time. Try to make sure most of the movement takes place below the elbow. Your shoulder should not move very much. All movement should be *slow* and *gentle*.

This exercise should be continued regardless of the advanced exercises you do.

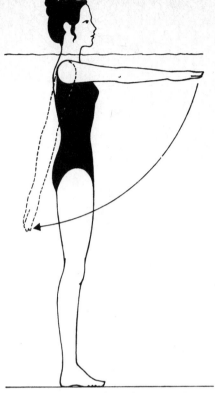

Exercise 7 — To *relax*, *stretch* and *strengthen* the muscles surrounding your shoulder joints.

Stand in water to midneck. Raise and lower your arm so that on the raising and lowering motions you feel as if you are *lifting* the water up and *pushing* the water down. All movement should be *slow* and *gentle*.

This exercise should be replaced with Exercises 34 and 35 as soon as you are able to do so.

This exercise does not put your shoulder through its full range of motion, which is achieved only when this exercise is replaced with advanced Exercise 34. Exercise 34 is the best way of putting your shoulder through its first full range of motion.

If you cannot eventually do Exercise 34, then Exercise 7 may be modified to provide full range of shoulder motion. Stand in water to midneck and raise your arm above the water so that it is perpendicular to the water. Then lower your arm as shown in the drawing for Exercise 7.

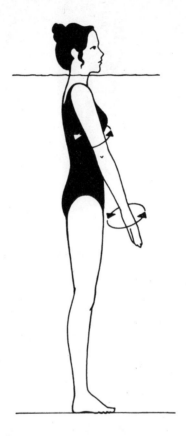

Exercise 8 — Further to *relax, stretch* and *strengthen* the muscles surrounding your shoulder joints.

Stand in water to midneck. Rotate your arms so that you feel as if you are *pushing* the water around in a narrow circular motion. Rotation should be to the right for a period of time and then to the left for a period of time. All movement should be *slow* and *gentle*.

This exercise should be replaced with Exercises 34 and 35 as soon as you are able to do so.

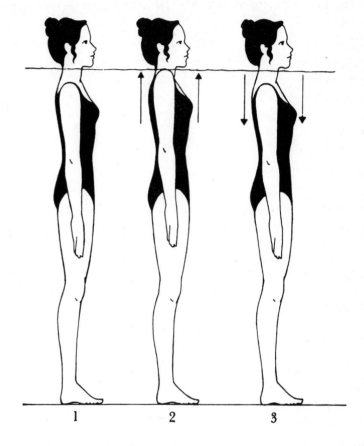

1   2   3

Exercise 9 — To *relax, stretch* and *strengthen* the muscles surrounding your lower-neck, upper-back and shoulder joints.

Stand in water to midneck. Raise and lower your shoulders in a shrugging motion. The raising motion should feel as if you are *pushing* the water up. All movement should be *slow* and *gentle*.

This exercise should be replaced with Exercise 10 as soon as you are able to do so.

Do these exercises for as long as you comfortably can without their becoming a strain. When you become tired, it is important that you stop and rest. After resting, repeat the exercise if you can.

In the beginning, if you can't even do any or all of these exercises for very long, or if you don't have the full range of movement pictured, it is important to have patience with yourself. In time your stamina and flexibility will increase naturally, and it will become much easier to do each exercise for longer periods of time with a greater radius of movement. The rule is always to try to do a little more than you did the last time, if you can do it without increasing the strain on yourself.

There is almost no benefit from doing these exercises once or twice a week. They should be done at least five times a week at the beginning. Then, once you have achieved your desired results, you can reduce to a three-times-a-week maintenance programme. Remember, results take time.

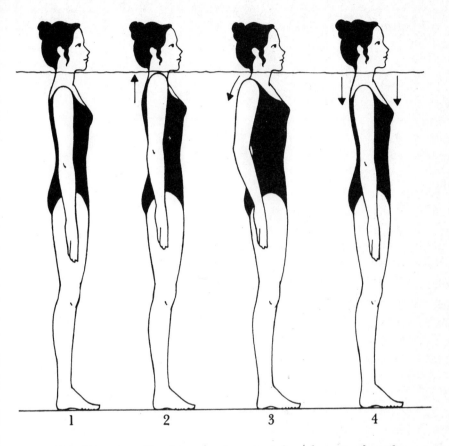

1   2   3   4

Exercise 10 — Further to *relax, stretch* and *strengthen* the muscles surrounding your lower-neck, upper-back and shoulder joints.

Stand in water to midneck as shown in Figure 1. Raise your shoulders straight up as shown in Figure 2. Then rotate your shoulders with a backward circular motion and start lowering them as shown in Figure 3. Return to starting position as shown in Figure 4. The raising motion should feel as if you are *pushing* the water up. All movement should be *slow* and *gentle*.

This exercise should be replaced with Exercises 34 and 35 as soon as you are able to do so.

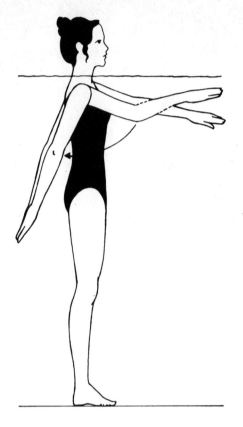

Exercise 11 — Further to *relax, stretch* and *strengthen* the muscles surrounding your shoulder, lower-neck and upper-back joints.

Stand in water to midneck. Move your arms up and around in front of you so that you cross your elbows. Then move your arms as far back behind you as they will comfortably go. All arm motion should feel as if you are *pushing* the water forward and backward. All movement should also be *slow* and *gentle*.

This exercise should be replaced with Exercises 34 and 35 as soon as you are able to do so.

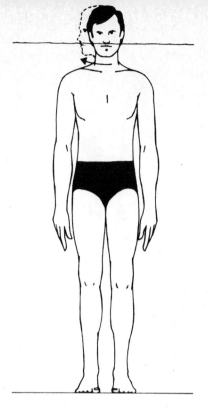

Exercise 12 — To *relax, stretch* and *strengthen* the muscles surrounding your neck joints.

Stand in water just below your nose. Keep your mouth closed and breathe through your nose. It is important that you stand in water this deep so that the water will be able to support your neck. Turn your head as far as you comfortably can to the right and then return to centre. Then repeat the same movement to the left. All movement should feel as if you are *pushing* the water. All movement should also be *slow* and *gentle*.

This exercise should be continued regardless of the advance exercise you do.

When doing this exercise be especially careful. If you feel the least bit dizzy, stop immediately. If you are in any way hesitant about being able to do the exercise safely, don't do it. Instead, concentrate on doing the lower-neck, upper-back and shoulder exercises, especially Exercises 10 and 11. Most of the neck muscles are connected to the upper back and the shoulders, and they can be successfully treated by effectively exercising those areas.

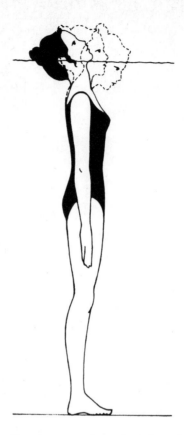

Exercise 13 — Further to *relax*, *stretch* and *strengthen* the muscles surrounding your neck joints.

Stand in water just below your nose. Keep your mouth closed and breathe through your nose. It is important that you stand in water this deep so that the water will be able to support your neck. Lower your head as far as it will comfortably go toward your chest. Then raise it as far back as it will comfortably go. All raising and lowering motions should feel as if you are *pushing* the water down and *lifting* the water up. All movement should be *slow* and *gentle*.

This exercise should be continued regardless of the advanced exercises you do.

NOTE: The warning for the preceding exercise (page 47) applies to this one too.

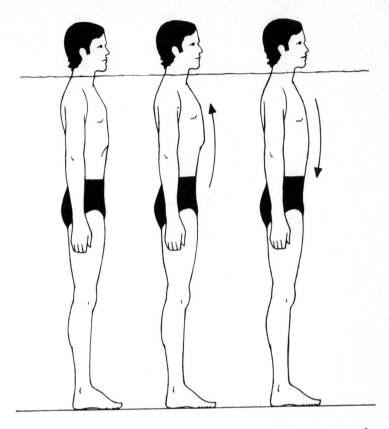

Exercise 14 — To *relax*, *stretch* and *strengthen* the muscles surrounding your upper-back joints and to improve your posture.

Stand in water to midneck. Breathe in deeply, raising your chest. Hold the chest up, then exhale. All movement should be *slow* and *gentle*.

This exercise should be replaced with Exercises 34 and 35 as soon as you are able to do so.

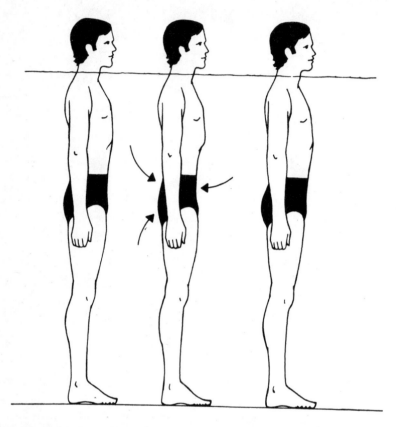

Exercise 15 — To *relax*, *stretch* and *strengthen* the muscles surrounding your lower-back joints and to improve your posture.

Stand in water above your shoulders. Tighten your buttock muscles and pull in your stomach, then release. All movement should be *slow* and *gentle*.

This exercise should be replaced with Exercises 34 and 35 as soon as you are able to do so.

Do these exercises for as long as you comfortably can without their becoming a strain. When you become tired, it is important that you stop and rest. After resting, repeat the exercise if you can.

In the beginning, if you can't even do any or all of these exercises for very long, or if you don't have the full range of movement pictured, it is important to have patience with yourself. In time your stamina and flexibility will increase naturally, and it will become much easier to do each exercise for longer periods of time with a greater radius of movement. The rule is always to try to do a little more than you did the last time, if you can do it without increasing the strain on yourself.

There is almost no benefit from doing these exercises once or twice a week. They should be done at least five times a week at the beginning. Then, once you have achieved your desired results, you can reduce to a three-times-a-week maintenance programme. Remember, results take time.

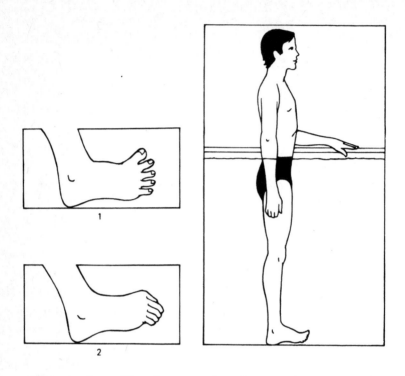

Exercise 16 — To *relax, stretch* and *strengthen* the muscles surrounding your toe joints.

Stand in water to your waist as shown. Hold on to the side of the pool. Stretch out and open your toes as much as you can as shown in Figure 1. Then attempt to clench them together as shown in Figure 2. All opening and closing motions should feel as if you are *pushing* the water forward and backward. All movement should be *slow* and *gentle*.

If you intend to do the exercise at home, see the caution on page 80.

This exercise should be continued regardless of the advanced exercises you do.

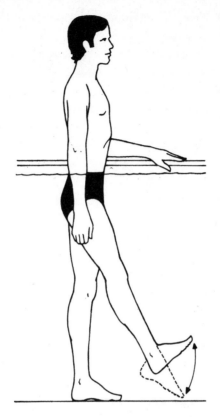

Exercise 17 — To *relax, stretch* and *strengthen* the muscles surrounding your ankle joints.

Stand in water to your waist. Hold on to the side of pool. Raise and lower your foot below the ankle so that on the raising and lowering motions you feel as if you are *lifting* the water up and *pushing* the water down. All movement should be *slow* and *gentle*. (At no point should your toes touch the floor.)

If you intend to do the exercise at home, see the caution on page 80.

This exercise should be continued regardless of the advanced exercises you do, though you do get partial benefit from Exercises 26 and 33.

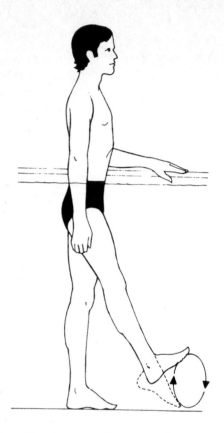

Exercise 18 — Further to *relax, stretch* and *strengthen* the muscles surrounding your ankle joints.

Stand in water to your waist. Hold on to the side of the pool. Rotate your foot below the ankle so that you feel as if you are *pushing* the water around in a circular motion. The direction of rotation should be to the right for a period of time and then to the left for a period of time. All movement should take place in your foot below the ankle. Try not to move your upper leg around. All movement should be *slow* and *gentle*. (At no point should your toes touch the floor.)

This exercise should be continued regardless of the advanced exercises you do.

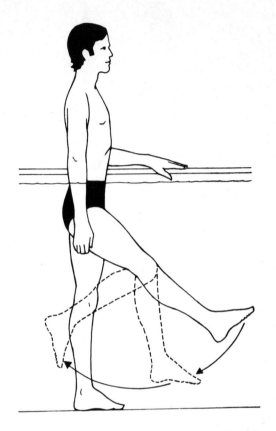

Exercise 19 — To *relax, stretch* and *strengthen* the muscles surrounding your knee joints.

Stand in water to your waist. Hold on to the side of the pool. Move your leg below the knee forward and backward so that you feel as if you are *pushing* the water forward and backward. All movement should be *slow* and *gentle*.

If you also have ankle problems, do the exercise the way it is described in Exercise 26. If not, then continue this exercise the way it is described here regardless of the advanced exercises you do.

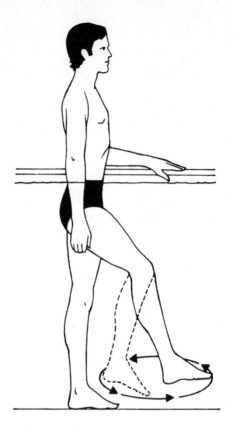

Exercise 20 — Further to *relax, stretch* and *strengthen* the muscles surrounding your knee joints.

Stand in water to your waist. Hold on to the side of the pool. Rotate your leg below the knee in a circular motion. The direction of rotation should be to the left for a period of time and then to the right for a period of time. Try to make sure that most of the movement takes place in your leg below the knee. Try not to move your upper leg around. All lower-leg movement should feel as if you are *pushing* the water. All movement should be *slow* and *gentle*.

This exercise should be continued regardless of the advanced exercises you do.

Do these exercises for as long as you comfortably can without their becoming a strain. When you become tired, it is important that you stop and rest. After resting, repeat the exercise if you can.

In the beginning, if you can't even do any or all of these exercises for very long, or if you don't have the full range of movement pictured, it is important to have patience with yourself. In time your stamina and flexibility will increase naturally, and it will become much easier to do each exercise for longer periods of time with a greater radius of movement. The rule is always to try to do a little more than you did the last time, if you can do it without increasing the strain on yourself.

There is almost no benefit from doing these exercises once or twice a week. They should be done at least five times a week at the beginning. Then, once you have achieved your desired results, you can reduce to a three-times-a-week maintenance programme. Remember, results take time.

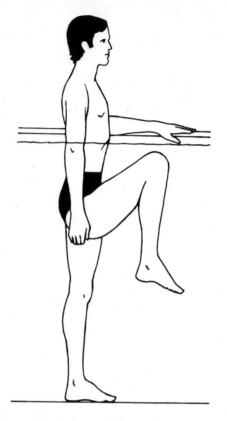

Exercise 21 — To *relax, stretch* and *strengthen* the muscles surrounding your knee, hip and lower-back joints.

Stand in water to the middle of your rib cage. Hold on to the side of the pool. Raise and lower your knee so that the raising and lowering motions feel as if you are *lifting* the water up and *pushing* the water down. All movements should be *slow* and *gentle*.

This exercise should be replaced with Exercises 32 and 33 as soon as you are able to do so.

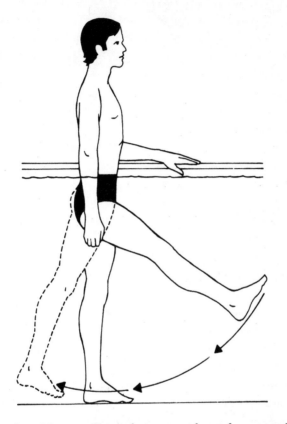

Exercise 22 — To *relax*, *stretch* and *strengthen* the muscles surrounding your hip joints, and straighten the muscles supporting your knee joints.

Stand in water to mid waist. Hold on to the side of the pool. Raise your leg forward, then lower it behind you, so that you feel as if you are *lifting* the water up and *pushing* the water down. All movement should be *slow* and *gentle*.

This exercise should be replaced with Exercises 32 and 33 as soon as you are able to do so.

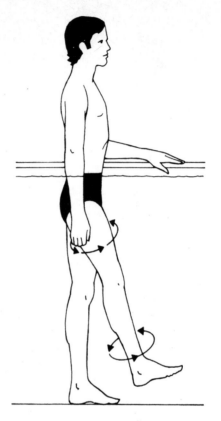

Exercise 23 — Further to *relax, stretch* and *strengthen* the muscles surrounding your hip joints.

Stand in water to midwaist. Hold on to the side of the pool. Rotate your leg so that you feel as if you are *pushing* the water around in a narrow circular motion. The direction of rotation should be to the right for a period of time and then to the left for a period of time. All movement should be *slow* and *gentle.*

This exercise should be replaced with Exercises 32 and 33 as soon as you are able to do so.

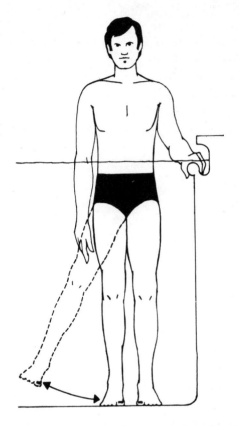

Exercise 24 — Further to *relax, stretch* and *strengthen* the muscles surrounding your hip joints.

Stand in water to midwaist. Hold on to the side of the pool. Raise and lower your leg sideways so that on the raising and lowering motions you feel as if you are *lifting* the water up and *pushing* the water down. All movements should be *slow* and *gentle*.

This exercise should be replaced with Exercise 31 as soon as you are able to do so.

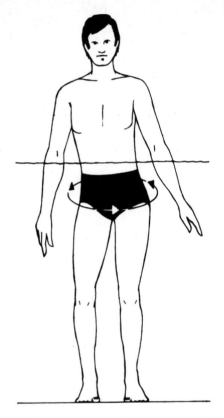

Exercise 25 — To *relax*, *stretch* and *strengthen* the muscles surrounding your hip and lower-back joints.

Stand in water above your waist. Rotate your hips so that you feel as if you are *pushing* the water around in a circular motion. Rotation should be to the right for a period of time and then to the left for a period of time. All movements should be *slow* and *gentle*.

This exercise should be replaced with Exercises 34 and 35 as soon as you are able to do so.

6 Intermediate Exercises

Intermediate and advanced exercises are especially beneficial to people who have arthritis pains in more than one area. They enable you to exercise different areas at the same time and thus spend more time on each area. For instance, Exercise 27 combines three beginner's exercises for your wrist, elbow and shoulder. Instead of spending ten minutes exercising your wrist, ten minutes exercising your elbow, and ten minutes exercising your shoulder, you can exercise all three for thirty minutes by doing this one exercise for thirty minutes. Most other intermediate and advanced exercises don't look like exact combinations of beginner's exercises, but your benefits from doing them are the same as from doing groups of beginner's exercises.

You can start doing intermediate and advanced exercises whenever you feel you have improved to the point where you are able to do them.

The first time that you do Intermediate Exercises involving floating and/or swimming be sure that you do them in shallow water. Some people are less buoyant than others. You probably won't have any problem, but if you should have trouble staying afloat, do not strain yourself to do so. Do not thrash around trying to keep yourself from sinking. Instead, the next time you exercise, wear one of the swimming aids described in the chapter on Exercise Aids. If you need a swimming aid to exercise comfortably do not be embarrassed about it. Remember that its purpose is to help you help yourself.

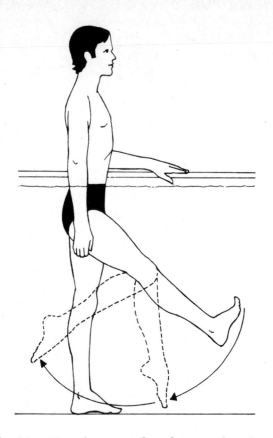

Exercise 26 — To *relax, stretch* and *strengthen* the muscles surrounding your ankle and knee joints.

Stand in water to your waist. Hold on to the side of the pool. Start with your leg raised and your foot below the ankle arched as far back as it will comfortably go. Then start to move your leg below the knee backward, at the same time pushing downward with the ball of your foot. Move your leg below the knee as far back as it will comfortably go and your foot below the ankle as far down and back as it will comfortably go. On the return upward motion raise both your leg below the knee and your foot below the ankle. All movement should feel as if you are *pushing* and *lifting* the water. All movement should also be *slow* and *gentle*.

This exercise should be continued regardless of the advanced exercises you do.

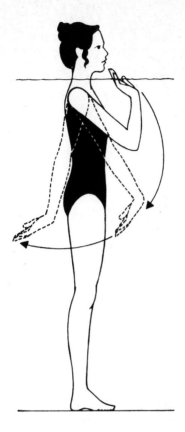

Exercise 27 — To *relax, stretch* and *strengthen* the muscles surrounding your wrist, elbow and shoulder joints.

Stand in water above your shoulders. Raise your arm and bend back your wrist as if you were a waiter carrying a tray. Then push down with both your arm and your hand below the wrist. Move them both as far back and down as they will comfortably go. On the return upward motion raise both your arm and your hand below the wrist. All movement should be *slow* and *gentle*. On all raising and lowering motions, you should feel as if you are *lifting* the water up and *pushing* the water down.

This exercise should be replaced with Exercise 32 and 33 as soon as you are able to do so.

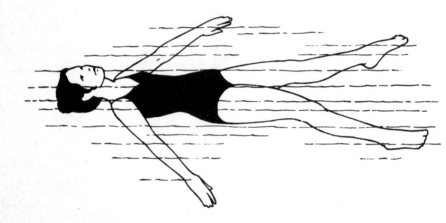

Exercise 28 — Floating isn't really an exercise in and of itself, but it is an excellent way to relax while you are resting between exercises. When you are floating, the water nestles under every curve of your body, thus giving your body total support. The floating position is also the base from which you can do many beneficial back and neck exercises. When floating, it is important to keep your toes pointed, your chest out, your back arched and your head back. If you have trouble floating, try spreading your legs wider apart to give yourself additional balance. If doing that doesn't enable you to float effortlessly, then you should wear a swimming aid.

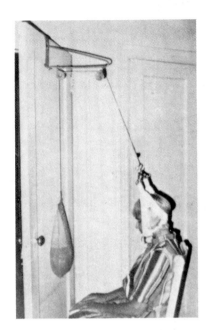

This is the type of over-the-door traction I did for years prior to my hospitalisation in 1972. The bag is filled with ten pounds of water. I used to sit with this weight pulling my neck for fifteen minutes at a time, three times a day. The supposed purpose of doing this was to stretch my neck muscles. In actuality this was slow torture to achieve little or no improvement.

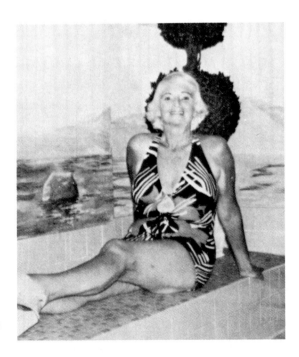

This is how I am today.

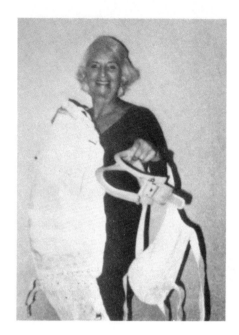

Now I no longer have to wear these monstrosities. In my right hand I'm holding the surgical corset I wore around my lower back. In my left I'm holding the collar I wore around my neck. Draped over my left arm is the back support I wore around my upper back. That was my third cervical collar, incidentally: I wore out the other two.

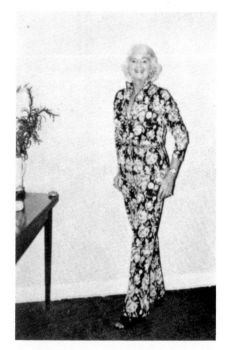

It's nice to be able to wear a dress like this without having to wear a cervical collar.

The best thing about this picture is that I'm standing straight. That doesn't seem like much, but standing straight was something I was unable to do for quite a few years.

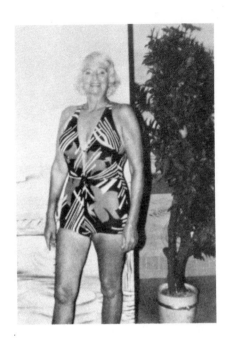

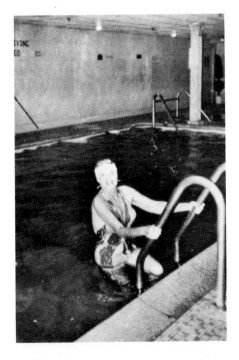

Contrary to some rumours there are times when I get out of the swimming pool.

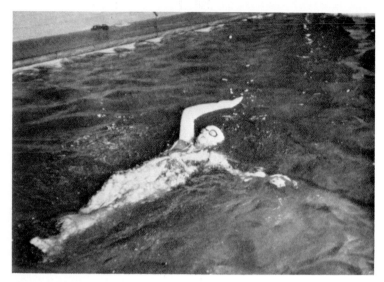

Exercise 34 is my modification of the conventional Olympic-style backstroke, which is designed for maximum speed. Mine is designed for maximum pain relief to the back and neck.

This is the whirlpool at an indoor health club. Remember that whirlpools are a pleasant luxury, not a necessity, but if you do use one you won't be smiling if you stay longer than three minutes.

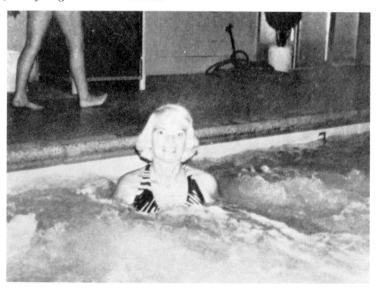

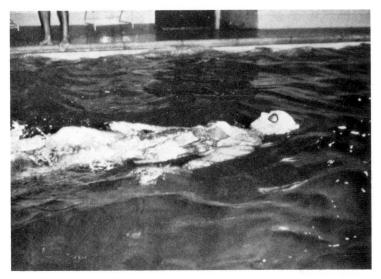

*I call this Exercise 35 'the wiggle'. When I do it for forty-five minutes,
swimming most effortlessly, I move each of my shoulders, arms, legs and hips
approximately 2,200 times.*

*This is Exercise 31. To receive the greatest benefit from it, be sure your arms
and legs do not merely skim the water. They should push the water forcefully,
first toward you and then away from you.*

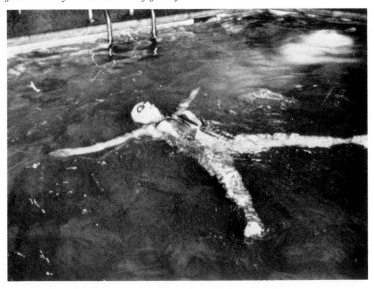

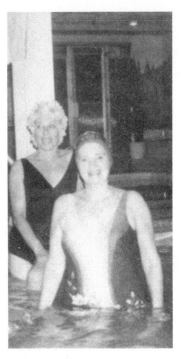

The woman in this picture is Gilda Bass. She has suffered from arthritis for many years and for the last fifteen of those years she had to sleep in a neck brace. A year ago, her condition was further complicated by an accident that caused a severe fracture and dislocation of her arm. Standard physiotherapy did not help her and she was told by her doctor that she would never be able to raise her arm again. She now no longer needs a cervical collar and she can lift her arm with ease.

With me is Al Mullarkey. In 1946 he injured his shoulder playing football and subsequently suffered with shoulder pain for over thirty years. Two years ago he also developed osteoarthritic pain in his hips and lower back. Today, as a result of proper water exercise he is pain-free.

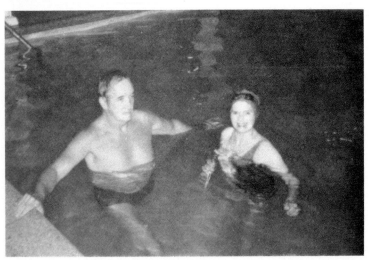

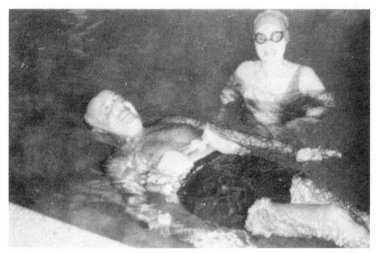

As a result of seven years of arthritis Leo Hase, pictured here, has partial bone fusion in his neck. A year ago Leo was taking liquid aspirin plus four Darvon (a pain killer) and four Motrin (an arthritis drug) a day for his pain. Additionally, he was unable to move his neck at all. He is now totally off Darvon and Motrin (though not yet off aspirin) and able to move his neck twenty-five degrees in each direction.

For the last five of his seventy-two years, Dave Herman, pictured here, suffered from arthritis of the hips and knees. Prior to starting water exercises he walked with a limp and was told by his doctors that he would either have to learn to live with the pain or submit to a hip-replacement operation. Today, as a result of water exercise, Dave no longer walks with a limp and is no longer in pain.

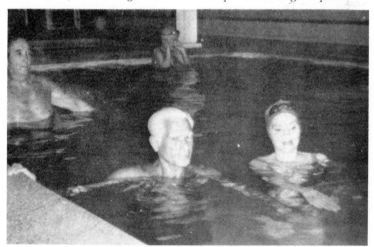

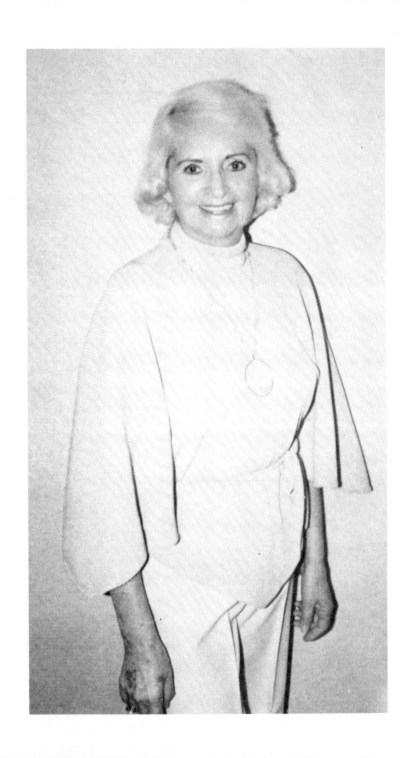

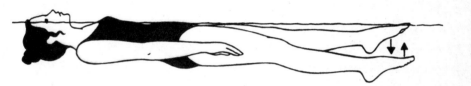

Exercise 29 — To *relax, stretch* and *strengthen* the muscles surrounding your lower-back, hip, ankle and knee joints.

In the floating position, with your arms at your sides and your legs close together, raise and lower your legs with a kicking motion. Your range of motion should be approximately eight inches, with your toes rising no more than an inch or two out of the water. All raising and lowering motions should feel as if you are *lifting* the water up and *pushing* the water down. All movement should be *slow* and *gentle.*

This exercise should be replaced with Exercise 35 as soon as you are able to do so.

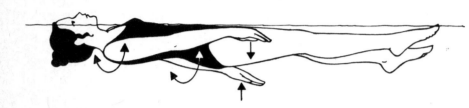

Exercise 30 — To *relax, stretch* and *strenghen* the muscles surrounding your neck, shoulder and upper-back joints.

In the floating position, with your arms at your sides and your legs close together, raise and lower your arms. Your range of arm motion should be approximately eight inches, with your arms never rising above the water. Your right arm should move downward as your left arm moves upwards. Then your right arm should move upwards as your left arm moves downward. The alternate up and down arm movement should give a natural twisting motion to your shoulders and your hips. This twisting motion is so beneficial you should try to encourage and exaggerate it. All raising and lowering motions should feel as if you are *lifting* the water up and *pushing* the water down. All movement should be *slow* and *gentle*.

This exercise should be replaced with Exercise 35 as soon as you are able to do so.

7 Advanced Exercises

Don't worry if you can't do the advanced exercises exactly the way they are drawn. I've been doing them for years and I'm not sure I do them exactly the way they are drawn. Realise that you will benefit greatly from doing them approximately right. The important thing is that you start doing them and then attempt to improve gradually.

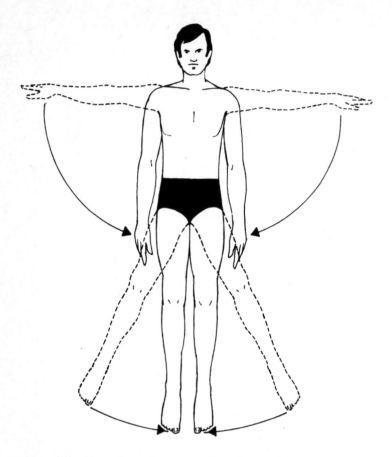

Exercise 31 — To *relax, stretch* and *strengthen* the muscles surrounding your shoulder and hip joints.

In the floating position, with your arms and legs extended, bring your arms down to your sides and your legs together. All movement should feel as if you are *pushing* the water. All movement should also be *slow* and *gentle*.

Don't mistake this for a standing exercise. The illustration shows an overview looking down on someone floating in the water.

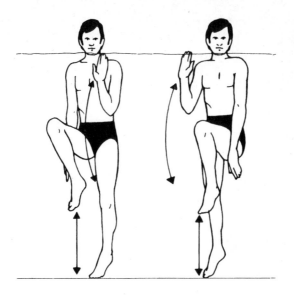

Exercise 32— To *relax, stretch* and *strengthen* the muscles surrounding your ankle, knee, hip, wrist, elbow, shoulder and lower-back joints.

This exercise is best done treading water in water over your head. If being in water over your head frightens you, start in water up to your chin. Raise and lower your knees, at the same time raising and lowering your arms below the elbows and hands below the wrist. Keep your wrists and ankles loose so that they get maximum up-and-down movement. The arm movement pictured here was purposely changed from the movement shown in swimming books, in order to give greater benefit to your wrists, elbows and shoulders. If you have lower-back pains, try to raise your knees as high as possible so as to achieve maximum stretching in your lower back. All movement should feel as if you are *lifting* the water up and *pushing* the water down. All movement should also be *slow* and *gentle.*

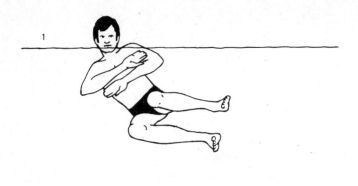

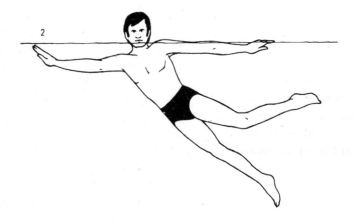

Exercise 33 — To *relax, stretch* and *strengthen* the muscles surrounding your wrist, elbow, shoulder, ankle, knee and hip joints — doing the sidestroke.

This isn't the classic sidestoke as taught in swimming books, but doing it this way gives added benefit to your wrists and elbows. On your side, cross your arms parallel in front of you and bring your knees up towards your stomach. Move your arms and legs outward, with your last outward movement being felt in your wrists and ankles. All movement should feel as if you are *pushing* the water. All movement should also be *slow* and *gentle*.

I find this exercise so relaxing that I sometimes do it for a few minutes as a rest in between my other exercises.

Exercise 34 — To *relax*, *stretch* and *strengthen* the muscles surrounding your neck, shoulder, back, hip, knee, ankle, elbow and wrist joints — doing the backstroke.

The twisting motion of the arms, the upper back and the hips pictured here is deliberately incorrect in terms of perfect swimming form (see below and pages 74-75). That is because your goal in doing this exercise is not to set Olympic swimming records but rather to provide maximum benefit to your neck, shoulders, back and hips. The additional twisting is the very thing that helps achieve that goal. It also enables you to move your elbows and wrists out of the water with minimum discomfort.

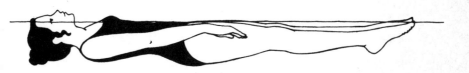

Figure 1: Start in the floating position with your hands by your sides and your legs close together.

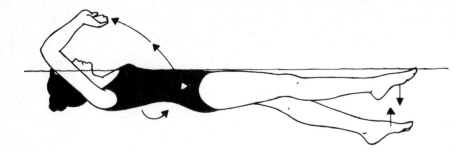

Figure 2: Start your kicking motion. Then raise your right arm backward so that the back of your right wrist passes over the left side of your head. On this raising motion you should both bend your elbow to the left and move your shoulder to the left. Your upper arm should almost touch your right ear as it passes near it. As your upper arm moves to the left your hips should twist slightly to the right.

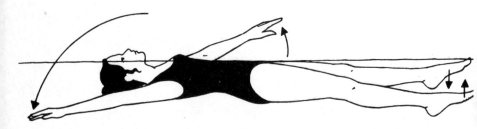

Figure 3: Continue kicking. Start raising your left hand out of the water. Rotate your right shoulder and wrist so that on your backward downward motion your palm faces the water and your fingers enter it first.

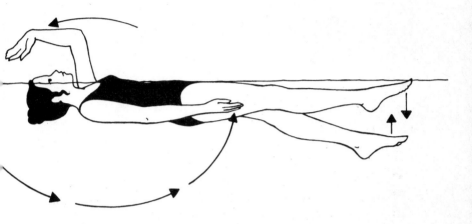

Figure 4: Continue kicking. Pass the back of your left wrist over the right side of your head. As your left arm moves up and to the right your hips should twist slightly to the left (not shown). Bring your right arm around through the water back to its original starting position. Your right arm is now in the starting position except that your palm is facing up instead of down. On each succeeding raising motion twist your wrist so that the back of your wrist can pass over the left side of your head.

All arm and leg movement should feel as if you are *pushing* and *lifting* the water. All movement should also be *slow* and *gentle*.

With this exercise, unlike Exercise 35, the more you twist your hips the more difficult it becomes to kick your feet. Both are beneficial, so try to find a happy medium between the two.

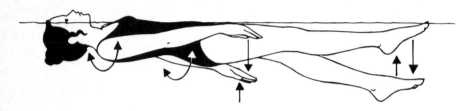

Exercise 35 — To *relax*, *stretch* and *strengthen* the muscles surrounding your neck, shoulder, back, hip, knee and ankle joints.

In the floating position, with your hands by your sides and your legs close together, raise and lower your arms and legs. The range of motion of your arms and legs should be approximately eight inches, with your toes rising no more than an inch or two out of the water and your arms never leaving the water. Your right arm and right leg should move downward as your left arm and left leg move upward. Then your right arm and right leg should move upwards as your left arm and left leg move downward. The alternate up-and-down movement should give a natural twisting motion to your hips and your shoulders. This twisting motion is so beneficial you should try to encourage and exaggerate it. All raising and lowering motions should feel as if you are *lifting* the water up and *pushing* the water down. All movement should also be *slow* and *gentle*.

The advanced exercises you find most beneficial will depend upon your particular condition. Personally, I find this exercise the most relaxing and pleasant one that I do. I use it to propel myself from one end of the pool to the other. I find this movement delightful.

ADVANCED-EXERCISE PROGRAMMES

My own advanced-exercise programme consists of forty-five minutes of alternating between Exercises 34 and 35. Then three minutes in the whirlpool, where I do the finger-flutter exercise, followed by forty-five more minutes of Exercise 34 and 35. In total, I usually do over 100 lengths of the pool, pausing only at the shallow end to clean my swimming goggles.

Occasionally, I also do sidestroke and water-treading exercises. I never do the crawl or the butterfly stroke, because doing them strains my neck and upper back. The reason for this is that in those strokes my neck and shoulders are above the water when I'm moving them.

I concentrate on Exercises 34 and 35 because they are the best advanced exercises for my condition. Between them, they are the best possible exercises for people whose main problems are hip, lower mid- and upper-back, shoulder and neck pains. If your main problems are with your wrists, elbows, ankles, knees, lower back and hips, the water-treading and sidestroke exercises are the ones you should spend most of your time doing.

In addition to the advanced exercises you do, if you have problems with your fingers or toes you will have to continue with the beginner's exercises for those conditions. Beginner's rotation exercises for ankles, knees, wrists and elbows should also be continued for a few minutes a day.

Even if you have arthritis pain in only one particular joint, it is still a good idea to spend some time doing a combination of advanced exercises. Any moderate exercise programme is good for your general health, and this one in particular will prevent arthritis pain from developing in other parts of your body.

Whether you suffer from single or multiple arthritis pains, you should continue to increase gradually the time you spend exercising, until you reach the point where you are no longer in pain. From the time I started doing beginner's exercises ten minutes a day altogether, it took me nine months to work my way up to one and a half hours and total freedom from pain.

Everyone's condition is different. You might progress much faster than I did or much slower. Regardless, wait until you are at least one month without pain before reducing your exercise frequency to four times a week. After being without pain for an additional month, you can reduce to the three-times-a-week minimum.

If you wish to be without arthritis pain, you must continue with your water exercises three times a week for the rest of your life.

I have reached the point where I no longer look upon these exercises as exercise. Aside from the physical benefits I have derived from them, I find them so pleasurable and relaxing that I have come to enjoy them for their own sake. I hope that once you have recovered, you will come to enjoy them as much as I do.

SUPPLEMENTAL HOME EXERCISE

There are some exercises that can be done beneficially at home to supplement your pool exercises. Exercises 1, 2, 3 and 4 may be done in a sink filled with water. Sit or stand, whichever is most comfortable for you. Do them as many times a day as you are able to do without straining yourself. If you find that sitting or standing this way out of the water strains any other part of your body, then confine your exercises to a pool. It is not worth it to worsen one condition to improve another.

Sink exercises plus Exercises 16, 17 and 18 may be done at home in the tub. I suggest you do them lying down so as not to chance slipping in the tub. If getting in and out of the tub is too much of a strain on your neck and back, do not attempt any of these tub exercises. I know the feeling, because for years I was in too much pain to take a tub bath.

If at all possible, these home exercises should be done in addition to pool exercises, not instead of them. Remember, beneficial advanced exercises cannot be done in a sink or bathtub.

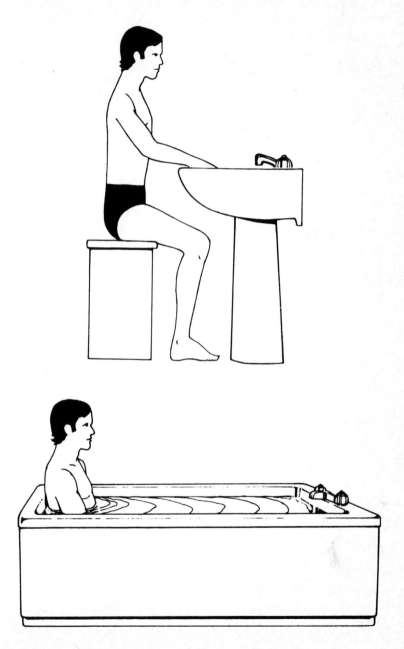

Exercising your hands and feet exclusively at home might not help. Your pain could be a referred pain. A referred pain is a pain felt in one part of the body but caused in another part of the body. It is possible that the pain in your hands is a referred pain caused by nerve pressure in your neck. The pain in your feet could also be a referred pain from your lower back. If that is the case, to get relief you must go to a pool and exercise the area that is causing your pain. For instance, if tense, tight and weak muscles press on nerve endings in your neck you might feel pain in your neck and also referred pain in your hands. If that is the case, then exercising your hands would not help your hands very much. To relieve both conditions you would have to go to a pool and exercise your neck.

Keep in mind that if you have pain in both your neck and your hands or lower back and feet one pain may be causing the other. If you have pain only in your hands or feet it is much less likely but still possible that the pain you feel is a referred pain. If you don't want to worry about referred pain, go to a pool and work up to doing advanced exercises.

8 Exercise Aids

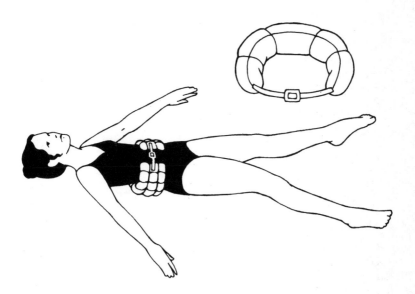

SWIM BELT*

If you are unable to float because you aren't naturally buoyant, this device will enable you to do so. Buckle the swim belt in front, just below your ribs. Relax and lie back on the water. You'll be amazed how easy it is to float. With the aid of a swim belt, you'll be able to participate in all the beneficial previously described exercises that start from the floating position.

*Also known as a water-skiing belt, see (8) page 96.

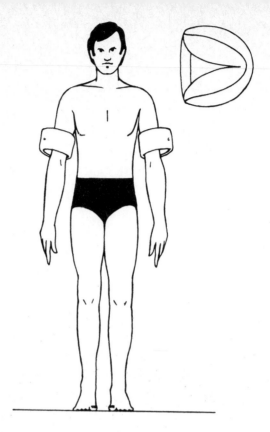

WATER WINGS*

This is an equally effective swimming aid of different design. Even though it is worn only on the upper arms it provides support for the entire body. If you aren't naturally buoyant or are afraid of the water these water wings will enable you to benefit from doing intermediate and advanced exercises that require the ability to float or swim.

Each wing has a flat side that is worn inward to allow for natural arm movement.

If you want this type of swimming aid drop me a note in care of my publisher (please enclose an addressed envelope with an appropriate International Reply-paid Coupon) and I'll be glad to supply a distributor's name.

*See (8) page 96.

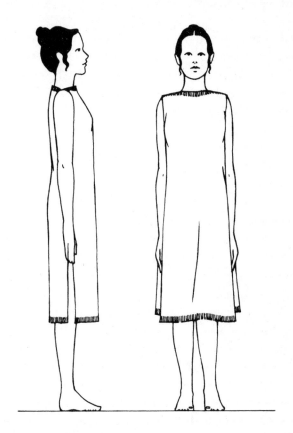

TURKISH-TOWEL TABARD

For use in the locker-room and going to and from the sauna and the shower in order to protect yourself from draughts, here is something you can put together yourself that is lighter to carry than a bathrobe and easier to put on.

To Make: Take two turkish bath towels and join two of the narrow ends, making sure that you leave an opening for your head to slide through easily.

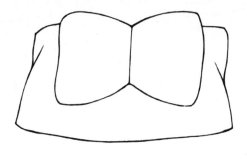

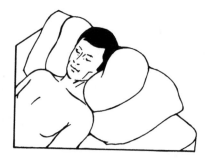

HOME-MADE CERVICAL PILLOW

If you need neck support when you are lying in bed, here is a tip that will save you the expense of buying a cervical pillow. Wrap ½ inch of elastic tightly around the middle of a regular pillow. Sew the ends of the elastic together. On top of another regular pillow, stand this pillow up on one of its longer sides and place your neck in the centre of the standing pillow. I have found this to give me better neck support than any cervical pillow that I ever purchased in a surgical-supply store.

9 My Life After

The pictures in this book indicate, I hope, that I am a real person. I don't have before-and-after pictures, because 'before' I didn't know there was going to be an 'after'. When I was sick and in pain I looked as bad on the outside as I felt on the inside and I wouldn't allow pictures of myself to be taken. All I can tell you is that people tell me that I look ten years younger now than I did five years ago.

Pain relief was the primary purpose of my special water exercise programme. An unlooked-for bonus is that in the last few years I've lost twenty pounds without dieting, firmed up my body and increased my energy level tremendously. I have also lowered both my pulse rate and my blood pressure.

I may be a little vain about my improvement, but the important thing is that my achievement is unique only because you haven't yet duplicated it. What I did you can do.

GENERAL COMMENTS ON MY RECOVERY

1. The feeling of accomplishment I have about my physical improvement makes me feel as if I were walking on water instead of exercising in water. Thinking about how crippled I was and how much better I am now because of my own efforts gives me a tremendous feeling of satisfaction and self-worth.

2. Everyone living on this earth has real and imagined problems that bother them. When mine start to get me down, I think about how much pain I used to be in, and that helps put whatever is bothering me in perspective.

3. Most drugs have unpleasant side effects (see Chapter 13). The pleasant side effects from my water exercises are that I've lost weight, firmed up and improved my figure and increased my general energy level. One can't imagine the

85

change in my attitude towards my body. I used to be so ashamed of my appearance, and now I feel so proud when the compliments roll in on how fit I look and how much stamina and endurance I now possess.

4. The important thing about my special water exercise programme is that it has enabled me once again to lead a normal functioning life. When I was sick, the acts of cooking, cleaning, walking, getting in and out of a car all caused me additional pain. Almost anything that required movement hurt me to one degree or another. Now, as long as I keep up with my water exercises, I can carry on all normal activities without any pain whatsoever.

5. When my arthritis first became serious, in addition to going to doctors, one of the first things I did was buy a book about arthritis. It took the doctor who wrote the book 170 pages to say 'Drink a lot of water, eat fruits and leafy green vegetables and think happy thoughts and your arthritis will go away'. It probably would have gone away if I had followed his advice and also coincidentally had a natural remission.

Before writing this book, I went to the library and read every book I could about arthritis to see if anyone else had discovered the benefits of water exercises. What I found amazed me. There were doctors saying that diet was the answer. Other doctors were saying not only that diet wasn't the answer, but that some of the diets were outright frauds. One doctor said massage was good for you, while another said it was harmful. The one I liked best was the doctor with a diagram of a neck exercise that could have easily killed a person with a neck a lot stronger than mine. The only reference I found to water treatment was the hospital use of the Hubbard Tank. This was said to be very beneficial to severely crippled arthritics.

6. I have heard many strange diets for arthritis. They range from adding zinc to your diet to drinking cod-liver oil to eating alfalfa seeds. According to the Arthritis Foundation, all of these exotic diets are just so much nonsense. The only type of diet they recommend is a normal well-balanced diet that should be eaten by everyone, whether they have arthritis or not.

My own experience confirms the opinion of the Arthritis Foundation. I have been eating the same foods during the period before I became sick, during the time I suffered most from arthritis and during my recovery. In those ten years, my condition changed drastically, but my diet remained the same.

7. One of the reasons people believe in quack cures is that at times they appear to work. People don't realise, though, that it is not the effectiveness of the 'cure' that's helping them but rather that they are having a natural remission from their arthritis. When and if these remissions occur, they occur regardless of the 'cure', not because of it.

It is unrealistic to expect a treatment to eliminate your pain unless that treatment effectively treats the cause of your pain.

8. When I was sick and in pain I couldn't stand the winter cold in New York. No matter how warmly I dressed, I felt stiffer and in more pain whenever I ventured outside. Now, as long as I dress warmly, the cold has no effect on me whatsoever.

9. When my hands were crippled, I had to shop for dresses that zipped down the front and bras that hooked in front. Now that I'm better, it is such a pleasure to look for clothes, worrying only if they are attractive, not whether I'm able to put them on or not.

10. I'll never forget when I was sick, bursting into a scream at some poor man who was just trying to be friendly. Upon being introduced, he shook hands with me before I could stop him. The pain in my hand was unbelievable, and his embarrassment at my reaction was even worse. I think of that incident now whenever I painlessly shake hands with new acquaintances.

11. Now that I'm no longer suffering, I have a much more positive outlook on life. I have a patience for people and an interest in doing things that I had found impossible when I was so involved in my own pain.

12. I've come a long way in my recovery. From not being able to hold a pen without pain, to being able to hold up a falling man. A friend of mine started to black out in

midsentence as we were standing beside the pool. I watched in horror as he started to fall slowly backward, head first, toward the tile floor. I grabbed him just in time with both my hands on his right arm, then quickly put my leg under him so that I could slide him to the floor without breaking his head. The strength of my grip on his arm was so great that he had ten black-and-blue marks that lasted for three weeks.

I hate to think what would have happened to this thirteen-stone man if my exercises hadn't strengthened my body to the point where I was able to help him.

13. To maintain my condition I only have to exercise three times a week, but when I have the benefit of a convenient pool I'll gladly swim seven days a week. When I find myself in a relatively empty pool I take advantage of the situation and swim for two or two-and-a-half hours instead of my normal one-and-a-half hours. I do this additional swimming because I really enjoy it.

After you have achieved your desired results you don't necessarily have to reduce to a three-times-a-week maintenance programme. If you have the time and you enjoy doing them, by all means continue your water exercises up to seven days a week for as many hours as you find pleasurable.

14. I don't want you to think that I've accomplished what I have because I'm some sort of superathlete. Before I started my special water exercise programme I hadn't exercised in forty years and I was additionally in a great deal of pain. I didn't start swimming a hundred lengths of the pool. When I started I couldn't do one length. Initially I had to work myself up to doing one width of the pool. All improvement just followed in natural slow progression. Once you start your programme you'll see for yourself how easy this really is.

15. When you are doing exercise to eliminate arthritis pain, the work ethic prevails. The more you do, the more you achieve. This special water exercise programme enables you to achieve more because it enables you to do more. If you were doing land exercise, you would have to torture yourself to build up to doing ten exercise repetitions. Once the pain factor is removed by exercising in water, there is almost no

limit to the number of repetitions you can gradually build up to doing.

During each maintenance session I do at least fifty lengths of the pool of Exercise 34 and at least fifty additional lengths of Exercise 35. In one length of doing Exercise 34 my arms, legs, shoulders and hips are each moved eight times. In one length of doing Exercise 35 my arms, legs, shoulders and hips are each moved forty-four times. In one hour-and-a-half session this adds up to moving each arm, leg, shoulder and hip 2,600 times.

These numbers shouldn't intimidate you. They should encourage you. Your buildup will be so gradual you won't realise you're doing it until you've done it. In fact, I had no idea I did so much until I counted for the purpose of writing this book. At any rate, swimming slowly on your back is effortless and pleasurable, not tortured and painful. When you compare the benefit derived from doing ten painful repetitions with the benefit from doing 2,600 painless ones, you can understand why my special water exercise programme is such a dramatic advance in the treatment of arthritis pain.

16. Throughout most of this book, I may sound self-inflated, but I don't think of myself as a heroine. I was terrified of my water exercises before I tried them, but I was even more terrified of becoming a complete cripple. So I tried.

The first time I ever went into a whirlpool, it took me seven days to get in. When I was told the temperature was 105 degrees, I was understandably wary. I decided to try it gradually. The whirlpool had four steps and I went in one step a day. Then I sat one minute the first day, two minutes the second day and finally three minutes the third day. It took me a week to finish a three-minute session. That's the way I've accomplished most of the things I've done. Nothing heroic, just slow, steady perseverence.

Preface to Part Two

Part Two of this book was written after Part One was published in the United States. The publication of Part One gave me the opportunity to see how well readers understood what I had written. Thus, I was able to note common mistakes and try to correct them in Part Two. Part Two consists of a re-emphasis of some important points made in Part One together with some additional information about water exercises, plus an overview of the standard medical treatments for arthritis. This overview is necessary for two reasons. First, to spur general change in the medical methods for treating arthritis. And second, to make you even more aware than ever of the importance, to you, of trying an alternative treatment such as water exercise.

10 The Three Factors That Make This Programme Work

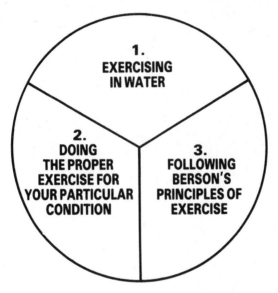

For this programme to work properly, you must faithfully follow all three parts of it. Few people have trouble with (1) and (2), but I have found that many people don't pay enough attention to (3). To avoid making this mistake, I suggest that you concentrate on making sure that you fully understand (3). In summary, the all-important 'principles of exercise' are:

(a) **Start with a level of exercise that you are comfortable with.**
(b) **Exercise regularly (five days a week).**
(c) **Without straining yourself gradually increase the amount of exercise that you are doing.**

(d) Over a period of months keep on increasing until you become pain-free.

(e) Once you have become pain-free, stay on a maintenance programme, at least three times a week, for the rest of your life.

The above is a brief summary. To understand everything fully, you should reread 24-35, 63, 77-8, 88-9 plus the new section on 'additional do's and don'ts'. Keep on rereading these pages until you have absorbed everything. If after doing that, you still have any questions, do not hesitate to write to me, care of my publisher with an addressed envelope and appropriate International Reply-paid Coupon.

ADDITIONAL DO'S AND DON'TS

1. You must keep on increasing the amount of exercise that you do until you become pain-free. I have discovered that some people achieve partial improvement by increasing the exercises up to a certain point and then stop increasing because they think that they have achieved all they can. This is a big mistake: the minimum exercise level required to make someone pain-free varies widely. Two hundred repetitions might be enough for one person and 2,000 might be required for someone else (in my case I needed the 2,600 exercise repetitions involved in doing a hundred lengths of the pool of Exercises 34 and 35. See (15) page 88. Thus, if you took two people who had gradually worked their way up to doing two hundred exercise repetitions, one might become pain-free and the other might feel only slightly better. Now, that does not mean that the second person cannot eventually become pain-free. It only means that he or she is not yet doing nearly enough exercise to make him or her pain-free.

There is no intelligent way to predict beforehand how much exercise will be necessary to make you pain-free. That is why you should not limit yourself to a set number of repetitions or a set amount of time devoted to exercise. What you must do is keep on increasing until you find the exercise level that is right for you.

2. Not increasing enough is the most common mistake people make. Less common, but just as serious, is trying to increase too rapidly. I know of a man who tried immediately to swim a hundred lengths of a pool because he read about the benefits that I got from doing so. One woman I know started doing one of the knee exercises, felt no pain, and then preceded to do one hundred repetitions. Needless to say, by the next day, both were in a lot of additional pain. And, needless to say, neither followed the correct procedure.

All increases must be gradual. The benefit from doing a hundred or a thousand repetitions does not come just from doing them. It comes from gradually working your way up to doing them. If you do things bit by bit then your muscles will gradually relax, stretch and strengthen. If you try to increase in a ridiculously fast manner then you will just wind up straining your muscles. Remember, the rule is not just to 'increase as much as you can'. The rule is to 'increase as much as you can without straining yourself'.

3. Incredibly, another mistake that some people make is that they don't pay adequate attention to the water level. Thus, I repeat again that you should always make sure that the water level is above the part of the body that you are exercising.

4. Prior to entering the pool, do not do warm-up exercises on land. In fact, you should not attempt any form of land exercise until you become pain-free. Once you become pain-free then you can determine for yourself what sports or activities may or may not be a strain on you.

5. Do not do any other forms of water exercise not shown in this book. While it is possible that one of the conventional swimming strokes (the crawl, etc) might help you somewhat, you would only be helped if part of your swimming movement accidentally coincided with the proper exercise for your particular condition. For best results, the safest and surest thing is to do nothing other than follow the programme exactly the way I have explained it to

you. I must also add a note of caution: if you suffer from back or neck pain, swimming on your stomach would not only be a waste of time, it would also be a strain on your back and neck.

6. Any physical strain that you put yourself under is going to slow down your recovery. That is why you should try to eliminate as much unnecessary strain as you can from your everyday activities. For instance, if you have leg pains, you should try to do much less standing and walking. If you have back, neck or arm pains, you should try to do much less pushing, lifting and carrying.

I realise that there are things that you have to get done that won't get done if you don't do them. But you must consider the physical consequences and weigh them against the importance of what you intend to do. That way you will be able to differentiate between what *should* be done and what *must* be done. When it comes to household- or job-related activities that may strain you, the idea is to eliminate everything that isn't absolutely necessary.

7. If you find that chlorine or other chemicals used in pool water irritate your eyes then you should wear swimming-goggles. Also, if you have allergies that affect your nose, you can wear nose-clips.

8. Most people, who have tried both, prefer the swimming belt to the water wings. So if you need a swimming aid, I suggest that you get the belt instead of the wings. Also, if you wish to purchase a swimming-belt, you should be aware that it is also, and sometimes more commonly, known as a 'water-skiing belt'.

9. Climbing down a ladder could strain you. So try to make sure that your swimming-pool has steps that you can use to walk into the water.

10. Do not be discouraged by bad days or weeks. People with arthritis sometimes experience particularly bad periods

when their pain is much worse than normal. It is possible that you might coincidentally go through a bad period during the first weeks and months that you are on the programme. If that happens, you shouldn't let a 'bad period' fool you into thinking that the programme isn't working for you. It *will* be working, but sometimes it takes a long time before it works so well that it can stop you from having temporary setbacks. What will happen though is that after you have been on the programme enough months your 'bad periods' will become less frequent and less severe until eventually they disappear entirely.

By the way, the definition of 'enough months' varies widely with the individual. Some people experience more or less continuous improvement from the beginning, while others experience temporary setbacks even after six months or more. Keep in mind that temporary setbacks are bound to happen. If they occur, just make sure that they don't discourage or deter you.

11 Improving the Quality of Life in Older Age

Obviously, eliminating pain is a major step towards improving the quality of life. Less obvious, but nevertheless important, are the other benefits that result from proper water exercise. The decline in ability to function (feelings of weakness, tiredness and listlessness that prevent you from doing nearly as much as you used to) that most people experience as they get older is an exaggerated, largely unnecessary decline. For the most part, this decline is not the natural result of 'old age', but the automatic result of too little use of the body.

Regardless of age, what you don't use will deteriorate. If a healthy twenty year old were confined to bed, after a month of confinement his legs, heart and lungs would all be measurably weaker. This wouldn't be weakness caused by 'old age' or disease, it would be weakness caused by disuse. And that is the type of weakness that most older people suffer from. As they get older they do less and less. And the less they do, the less able they become to do anything. Luckily for the mythical twenty year old and luckily for you, this type of decline is reversible.

One of the reasons that I emphasise the advanced exercises is that doing them properly (over a period of time, gradually increasing the number of laps you do) will greatly strengthen your heart and lungs. It is this improvement in the functional capacity of heart and lungs that makes people feel younger and more energetic. And it is this feeling of strength and energy that makes people better able to enjoy their lives in older age.

By the way, this type of improvement is not unique to water exercise. Sustained jogging, bicycle-riding and cross-country skiing have all been shown to produce similar strengthening of heart and lung capacity. The problem with these exercises though is that they also produce a degree of leg and body strain that makes them unsuitable for most older people and quite a few younger ones. The great advantage of proper water exercise is that it strengthens your heart and lungs without straining the rest of you.

12 Not All Water Exercise Programmes Are the Same

Most laymen have never previously heard of water exercise as a treatment for arthritis. And while most doctors have heard of it, many doctors are not aware of the specifics of various water exercise programmes. Thus, because of unfamiliarity, both groups have a tendency to assume that all water exercise programmes are the same, simply because they are all done in water. Upon close examination, this assumption makes as much sense as assuming that soccer, pole-vaulting and tennis are all the same, simply because they are all done on land.

Just as there are differences between various land exercises, there are great differences between my water exercise programme and the water exercise programmes currently carried on in most hospitals.

What the hospital programmes and my programme have in common is that some of my beginner's exercises are shared by both programmes. The first important difference is that the hospital programmes have nothing comparable to my intermediate and advanced exercises. But the major difference is in 'principles of exercise'.

Medical scientists have long understood that for drugs to be maximally effective they must be taken at the proper dosage and frequency. What I have discovered is that the same thing holds true for arthritis exercise. With insufficient dosage and frequency, arthritis exercise produces only minimal results, but with proper dosage and frequency it produces spectacular results.

In terms of frequency, exercising once or twice a week is

not enough to achieve progressive improvement. When you exercise that infrequently, whatever is gained from one exercise session is lost by the time the next session comes along. As I explained in the analogy on page 20, if you don't exercise often enough, you will always have to start over again at 100 units and you will never really improve.

While it is possible to achieve progressive improvement exercising three times a week, it is only barely possible. In terms of faster improvement and in terms of certainty of improvement, five times a week is much better.

As far as duration goes, I would not know how it is possible to decide the ideal exercise time. Everyone's condition is different. What is enough exercise to make one person pain-free isn't necessarily enough for another. Setting artifical time limits, of any sort, is equivalent to setting a limit on the degree to which you will allow yourself to recover. Instead, the intelligent way to do things is to keep on gradually increasing exercise duration until you become pain-free.

Because of the heat of the water and deficiencies in duration and frequency of exercise, some hospital pool programmes are in effect more like heat treatments than exercise programmes. The rationale for using very hot water is that heat temporarily relaxes the muscles, thus making it initially easier to exercise. The problem with very hot water is that the heat weakens you, thus making it impossible to exercise for long periods of time and thus depriving you of the benefits of extended exercise.

The people who run these hospital programmes believe that it is not possible for arthritics to exercise in water cooler than the high nineties. The fact is that most arthritics have no trouble whatsoever with exercising in normal pool temperatures of eighty to eighty-five degrees. And for the few who do feel some chill, all that has to be done is to start them out in hot water and then gradually lower the temperature as they warm up from moving around in the water. Since heat treatments provide temporary relief but no long-term benefit, and since gradually increased exercise results in progressive improvement, it is obvious that the emphasis of pool programmes should be much less on heat and much more on exercise.

In addition to insufficient duration and frequency and not doing the best exercises, these programmes compound their errors with a glaring omission. There is not one expert on exercise or arthritis who maintains that muscles remain in a constant state. They all agree that no matter how much you have improved your muscles by exercising them, that improvement lasts for only as long as you continue with the exercise programme. As soon as you abandon the programme your muscles start to deteriorate from disuse. That is why on my programme people are encouraged to continue with a maintenance level of exercise for the rest of their lives. And that is why it is inexcusable that other programmes make no such provision for lifetime maintenance.

Finances permitting, I would like to see all pool programmes altered to follow the principles of exercise that I advocate. I think that the great majority of arthritics can follow my programme without using a hospital pool. But for the others, who are too crippled to travel to a pool or too crippled to get in and out of a pool without assistance, a good hospital programme would be very beneficial for starting people out with water exercise. If the programme is good, it should only take a couple of months before most patients improve to the point where they can then follow the programme on their own in a public pool.

When I teach my programme I consider a class of one to be ideal and a class of two or three possible. I find that classes larger than three are unmanageable in terms of dealing with individual needs. Also, once people have learned the exercises and understand the proper 'principles of exercise', classes are unnecessary. Patients can then proceed on their own at a pace that is individually best for them.

When I started doing exercises for arthritis, there were other people at the health club who also suffered from arthritis. These other people would stand around in the water, dunk themselves, swim and/or do water calesthenics. By the time I had become pain-free, these people still had their pain. When I started to realise why I had accomplished what I had, I also started encouraging other people to follow my example. The first two people who listened also became pain-free. And soon quite a few more people started my programme and started to get better from it. Yet incredibly, there were and still are, some arthritics at the pool who won't listen. These people swim around in the same water as people who are pain-free and yet they are oblivious to the fact that they too could be helped.

My discussion of other people at my health club points out some interesting things about human nature, but of more importance is what it explains about water exercise. It is for this same reason of explaining water exercise that I have entered into a discussion of other water exercise programmes. My purpose was not to belittle or disparage them, but to emphasise an important point: 'Not all water exercise programmes are the same. Exercising in the water makes exercise much easier, but doing the proper exercises and following the proper "principles of exercise" is what makes you better.'

13 Arthritis and Drugs

In response to Federal law, in the US, pharmaceutical companies must make available to physicians and pharmacists a list of the adverse reactions of the prescription drugs that they manufacture. To prevent possible lawsuits, the drug manufacturers must be totally candid. The following lists of side effects were not copied from literature put out by anti-drug fanatics. They were copied directly from the literature that the drug companies themselves have printed and distributed in order to comply with the law. Below is a partial listing of the side effects these drugs cause.

Prednison is a cortisone type drug used in the treatment of rheumatoid arthritis, and some of the other less-common forms of arthritis. Under 'adverse reactions' the manufacturer lists: sodium retention, fluid retention, congestive heart failure in susceptible patients, potassium loss, high blood pressure, muscle weakness, loss of muscle mass, osteoporosis, vertebral compression, fractures, pathologic fractures of long bones, peptic ulcer with possible perforation and haemorrhage, pancreatitis, abdominal distention, ulcerative, oesophagitis, impaired wound healing, thin fragile skin, increased sweating, convulsions, vertigo, headache, menstrual irregularities, suppression of growth in children, manifestations of latent diabetes mellitus, posterior subcapsular cataracts, increased intraocular pressure and glaucoma. Under 'precautions' the manufacturer states 'psychic derangements may appear when corticosteroids are used, ranging from euphoria, insomnia, mood swings, personality changes and severe depression to frank psychotic manifestations'. Many non-steroidal, anti-rheumatic agents are in common use, among them:

Indo methacin (Indocid): an anti-inflammatory drug used in the treatment of rheumatoid arthritis, osteoarthritis and other less common forms of the disease. Under 'warnings' the manufacturer states that 'single or multiple ulcerations, including perforations and haemorrhage of the oesophagus, stomach, duodenum or small intestine have been reported to occur with Indocin. Fatalities have been reported in some instances'. Under 'adverse reactions' the manufacturer lists nausea, indigestion, heartburn, diarrhoea abdominal pain, constipation, headache, dizziness, vertigo, depression and fatigue, anorexia, peptic ulcer, rectal bleeding, intestinal ulceration, gastrointestinal bleeding, psychic disturbances including psychotic episodes, mental confusion, drowsiness, rash and anaemia.

Diflunisal (Clinoril): an anti-inflammatory drug used in the treatment of osteoarthritis, rheumatoid arthritis and other forms of arthritis. Under 'warnings' the manufacturer states 'peptic ulceration and gastrointestinal bleeding have been reported in patients receiving Clinoril'. Under 'adverse reactions' the manufacturer lists the most common ones as being: gastrointestinal pain, nausea, with or without vomiting, diarrhoea, constipation, anorexia, gastrointestinal cramps, rash, itching, dizziness, headache and nervousness.

Fenoprofen (Fenopron) is an arthritis drug used in the treatment of osteoarthritis and rheumatoid arthritis. Under 'adverse reactions' the manufacturer lists the most common ones as being: indigestion, itching, drowsiness, ringing in the ears, heart palpitations and headache. Other 'adverse reactions' listed were: constipation, nausea, vomiting, abdominal pain and rash.

Naproxen (Naprosyn): a drug used in the treatment of rheumatoid arthritis and osteoarthritis. Under 'warnings' the manufacturer states 'gastrointestinal bleeding, sometimes severe, and occasionally fatal, has been reported in patients receiving Naprosyn'. Under 'adverse reactions' the manufacturer lists: heartburn, nausea, indigestion, abdominal pain, constipation, diarrhoea and vomiting.

The way I 'chose' these drugs was to ask my local druggist for the manufacturer's literature on the most commonly prescribed arthritis drugs. Of the eight drugs that his store stocked, he happened to have literature for five of them. That's how these five were chosen.

In terms of arthritis, a year or even three years must be considered to be a short term. People who have arthritis, and don't follow my programme, usually suffer from it for the rest of their lives. If they are given drugs for their pain, then they could wind up being dependent on drugs for ten, twenty or even thirty years. Amazingly, these lists of drug reactions have resulted from relatively short-term testing of one to three years. Not only that, but most of the patients involved were not even tested for the entire length of the clinical trials. For instance, one test involved 737 people but only 256 of them were given the drug for as long as two years. Another test involved 1,865 people, but only 232 of them were given the drug for at least forty-eight weeks.

So, unpleasant as these lists of 'adverse reactions' are and as harmful as these drugs can be, based on clinical testing, in actual long-term use, they are probably even worse for you. The manufacturers' lists and percentages do not tell you what taking these drugs for five or ten years will do to your body. Based on the manufacturers' figures, you can only guess at the actual damage that long-term use will cause.

What I find disturbing about all this is that most arthritics have no idea of the risks that they could be taking. The law mandates that doctors and pharmacists be informed, but says nothing about unsuspecting patients. A better law would require that patients be accurately informed of the dangers. The probability of each and every adverse reaction should first be fully determined. Then, this probability should be fully explained to patients in language that they can understand. Let an informed public decide whether or not taking arthritis drugs is worth the risk.

DANGEROUS AND INEFFECTIVE

The injection or occasional ingestion of drugs is by far the most common form of treatment for arthritis. Since these drugs can be dangerous to your general health, it would be logical to assume that the reason that they are used so much, in spite of the dangers, is that they are very effective. Unfortunately, sound logic has very little to do with the treatment of arthritis. In the US, arthritis drugs are being routinely prescribed in spite of their known limitations.

In reference to the effectiveness of these drugs, their 'benefits' vary with the individual. Some people experience a marked temporary reduction of pain. Others experience a slight reduction. And still others continue to feel worse regardless of the drugs that they take. What I mean by 'ineffective' is that no one experiences long-term benefits. These drugs will not make you feel progressively better. They will not eventually make you pain-free. While it is always possible that someone with arthritis could experience a natural remission, barring such good luck an arthritic faces the possibility of a lifetime of dependence on drugs.

If your doctor allows or encourages continued long-term

drug use, then two situations can develop. First, partially reduced pain may be paid for at the price of other diseases. Second, after a while the drugs could stop helping and you could wind up suffering from both terrible 'adverse reactions' and terrible arthritis pain.

Allowing for variations, that's basically the picture. It's not a pretty picture but it's the one that I've seen. Since there are no published statistics on the longer-term lack of effectiveness of arthritis drugs, I will explain how I've come to see things the way I do.

First, there was my own personal experience. While I did get twenty-five per cent relief from both cortisone and gold injections, that relief was only temporary. Over a six-year period, I continued to get worse each year, in spite of all the medical treatments that I received. In the light of what I now know about water exercise, I realise that my six years of physical suffering plus the thousands of dollars I spent on treatments, was all for nothing. The only thing that I'm thankful for is that I wasn't on drugs long enough to be permanently harmed by them. (Please note that just because I wasn't harmed by short-term exposure to drugs, that doesn't mean that you can't be. There is more involved than just the length of time you take these drugs. Also involved is your particular susceptibility to them.)

Second, I have had conversations with hundreds of long-term arthritics. I don't know whether all these people just happened to be malcontents, but almost none of them were satisfied. The most common complaints were objections to continued pain and the high cost of worthless medical treatments.

Third, I spoke to two pharmacists that I know. The first, talked about people 'burning holes in their stomachs'. I asked the second if in fifteen years in business he had seen anyone helped by arthritis drugs. He answered, 'On a short-term basis some people are helped, but long term, no one that I've seen.' An acquaintance of mine told me her pharmacist tells people, 'If you can stand the pain, you are better off not taking drugs.'

WHY DRUGS?

When you weigh their potential for harm against their potential for good, the obvious question is, 'Why drugs?' Why are doctors prescribing them and why are patients taking them? What in the world is going on here?

First, I'll discuss this from the patient's point of view. Ninety-nine per cent of patients have never heard of Dvera Berson and her water exercise programme. And many of those that have heard only a little about it, aren't interested. People in pain have a natural desire for instant solutions. And taking drugs fits in with that desire a lot more easily than does water exercise. What it comes down to is that almost no one knows that a better answer exists.

Also, when most patients start taking arthritis drugs, they are totally unaware of the dangerous side effects. And most of those few that are aware, aren't totally aware. They've heard that arthritis drugs 'can be bad for you', but they have never read the appropriate literature to find out exactly how bad these drugs really are. Additionally, many people start out with a misconception about the value of drug treatments. Because of major advances such as the advent of life-saving antibiotics, people have come to believe that there is an effective drug answer for everything. This results in people thinking that if they get sick, all they have to do is take the proper drug and soon they will be better. One day it may come to pass that there will be safe drug cures for everything. Unfortunately, medical science is still very far away from that ideal.

So, what we have is people who are unaware of the dangers and lack of effectiveness of drugs, who also want relief as soon as possible. This then combines with the most important factor that encourages people to take drugs, which is people's tendency towards blind faith in their doctors. Even though I don't think much of having blind faith in anyone human, I understand such faith because I once had it. As I have said, for six years I was an exceptionally dutiful and obedient patient. Only bitter

107

experience finally taught me to question and examine everything.

To understand why rheumatologists prescribe drugs so readily for arthritis, it is necessary to provide some background information about the attitude of most doctors (not just rheumatologists) towards drugs. Over the last thirty or forty years many life-saving drugs have been developed. These drugs have made doctors much more effective in their ability to fight disease. Thus, many doctors have come to think of drug treatments as being very beneficial. Diagnosis has become the first step in deciding which drug to use. Doctors want to diagnose a disease correctly so that they can then prescribe the best available drug. So far, so good. But, unfortunately, what this has all evolved into is that many doctors have come to think of drug treatments as 'the' method by which disease should be fought. Doctors have become so used to prescribing drugs for everything that they have difficulty imagining alternative treatments. Thus, for some diseases they routinely prescribe the best existing drug, with too little regard to how toxic and/or ineffective that drug may possibly happen to be.

Another factor that contributes to the over-prescription of drugs is the influence that the drug companies exert over doctors. These companies spend millions of dollars a year on medical advertising. Professional magazines abound with advertisements extolling the virtues of various drugs. In the US the drug companies also send around 'detail men' to speak to doctors who are in private practice. These 'detail men' act in a friendly, respectful manner and also give the doctors free drug samples. What they speak about are the virtues of the particular drugs that their company happens to be selling. With all this advertising and personal attention it is easy to see how even the most objective doctors could be somewhat seduced into viewing the world the way the drug companies do.

In spite of the aforementioned subtle and not so subtle influences, a case could still be made that most doctors' behaviour is correct within the limits of what they know. Specifically with arthritis, a case could be made that arthritis drugs are used' so extensively because doctors don't know what else to do and they are merely trying to do the best they can in difficult circumstances.

The difference between Britain and the United States is that in the US doctors profit financially from the treatments that they suggest. Medicine is practised on a fee-for-service basis. What that means is that the more patients a doctor sees and the more drugs and tests each patient is given, the more money the doctor makes. With a chronic disease such as arthritis, patients can turn into lifetime customers. They have to keep coming back for injections and/or prescriptions. And of course, they have to keep having their bodies tested for adverse drug reactions. With all this potential for profit, I don't think that it is a coincidence that most American rheumatologists just happen to see things the way the drug companies do.

Regardless of national variations in the profit motive, the situation that exists throughout the world is that the arthritis experts aren't very expert. Yes, there are many arthritis doctors who may be defined as 'experts' in terms of the medical degrees that they hold, and in the number of papers that they have had published and in the professional esteem of their colleagues. But in terms of their ability to actually help arthritis sufferers these 'experts' are sadly lacking in expertise.

What I would like to see is current arthritis treatments justified in terms of their effectiveness. I want to see the doctors try to do that. I don't think they can, but I would like to see them try. And when and if they do try, I think it would be a step forward if the doctors' statements were not blindly accepted as expert opinion. Instead, I would like to see their answers closely examined by an interested and informed public, press and government.

Of course, what I would really like to see is a great change in the direction and emphasis of arthritis care. There should be movement away from what is dangerous and ineffective and towards what is much more helpful. My ideas on this subject are more fully discussed in the chapter on 'the way things should be done'.

HOW TO GET OFF DRUGS

I believe that arthritis drugs can be dangerous and are often unnecessary. That is why I also believe that as you improve from water exercise, you should try to reduce and then eliminate your intake of arthritis drugs. If you agree with me and want to end your dependence on drugs, it is important that you do so in a safe and proper manner, in consultation with your doctor.

When getting off drugs the general idea is to try for gradual reduction. For instance, if you take a drug four times a day you shouldn't just stop taking it. Instead you should try taking it three times a day and see how you react to the reduction. If everything is fine, then after a week or two, you could further reduce to two pills a day. And then after another week or two to one. A drug that is taken once a day, could be reduced to three out of four days, then to two out of three days, then to every other day, then to one out of three days and then eliminated.

Make sure that each reduction that you make is the least possible reduction you can make. For instance, if you are taking ten pills a day your first reduction should be to nine pills, your second to eight and your third to seven etc. Also, make sure that after each reduction you maintain your new level for a week or two before you attempt to reduce it further.

'Slow and gradual' are the watchwords both for water exercise and drug elimination. This is true for all arthritis drugs and painkillers, but it is especially true for cortisone-type arthritis drugs. With any arthritis drug, reduction of dosage increases the possibility of increased discomfort from arthritis. But with cortisone there is the added possibility of experiencing withdrawal symptoms from the drug itself. Again, that is why I caution that drug reduction must be slow and gradual.

Aside from the dangers of rapid reduction, there are benefits from doing things slowly. If your reduction is gradual enough, it is possible that lower doses won't cause you any increased discomfort, because whatever benefit you would be losing from the drug would be gradually replaced by benefits from water exercises. To encourage this type of more-or-less painless drug reduction, a certain rule should be followed: 'If a reduction in your drug dosage causes you any increased discomfort, do not make another reduction until that increased discomfort has disappeared.'

Please note that I do not advocate the immediate reduction of drugs as soon as you start your water exercise programme. Most people experience no increased discomfort from starting their programme, but a few people do. This increased pain is a warning signal that you are either overdoing an exercise or doing an exercise that is wrong for your particular condition. Unfortunately, this increased pain doesn't always occur at the time that you are exercising. It may occur any time in the following forty-eight hours. Thus, if your drug reduction was simultaneous with starting water exercises, you wouldn't know whether your increased discomfort was caused by less drugs or by a correctable mistake that you are making in the pool. 'The idea is to first make sure you are doing everything right with your water exercise programme before you complicate things by lowering your drug intake.'

Also, for the purpose of maintaining high morale, I think it is important that you be totally confident of your water exercise programme. Getting off drugs and becoming painfree requires sustained effort for a long period of time. That is why I think that you should first establish a definite pattern of improvement from water exercise before you attempt to end your dependence on drugs. Once you have confidence that water exercise really works, then getting off drugs will not seem like such a big hurdle.

As much as I would like to, I can't tell you precisely how soon after you start your water exercise programme you should start your drug reductions. In absolute terms of weeks and months, it varies with the individual. But the right time for you is whenever you are sure that you are following the programme properly and that it is helping you. If you experience no increased discomfort from being on the programme, then you know that you are doing things properly. Once you start to experience a significant reduction in your pain then you know that the programme is working. At whatever point in time that happens, then that's the time to start ending your dependence on drugs.

Instead of bothering to write all of the above, I could have merely written, 'If you want to know how to get off drugs, ask your doctor.' My main reasons for not confining my remarks to that one sentence were: (1) doctors don't always have the time, or take the time, to explain things properly to their patients; (2) most doctors are not familiar with the intricacies of water exercises — much less the intricacies of water exercises as they relate to drug reduction; (3) since your doctor was probably the one to put you on drugs in the first place, he might feel professionally insulted that you, or I, are suggesting an alternative treatment.

Sitting here writing this book, I have no idea what your doctor may be like. He may be very competent and sympathetic or he may not. Assuming some degree of competence, then I must add that the best way for you to get off drugs is in co-operation with your doctor (keeping in mind everything I have written). Your doctor knows about, or he can look up, the pharmacology of the specific drugs that you are taking. And you are the expert on how your body is reacting to drug reductions. Between you both, you should be able to work out something beneficial.

14 Confusion over the Cause of Arthritis Pain

Most laymen are not aware of what causes arthritis pain. And those that are have difficulty accepting what they have learned. To set the record straight, I emphasise that the following is not just my theory. These are the facts: while no one yet knows what causes arthritis, the cause of arthritis pain has been indisputably established. It is medically accepted that arthritis involves deterioration of bones and joints, but tense, tight and weak muscles are the immediate cause of almost all arthritis pain.

Most doctors are aware of this fact, but nevertheless they don't seem to be totally aware. For instance, their knowledge has not inspired them to expend much thought or effort toward treating the muscular component. On a functional level they still think of arthritis pain exclusively in terms of bone and joint damage.

Ever since I started researching the subject of arthritis, I noticed that most doctors seemed to pay very little attention to treating this muscular component. It is only recently though that I have become aware of the mental dichotomy that is partially responsible for this situation. The way I became aware is explained by the following:

On a trip to the country I became involved in a minor automobile accident. As a precaution, I went to a local doctor. After examining my X-rays, he expressed great surprise that I wasn't in terrible pain. The doctor hadn't found any broken bones. Instead, what he found was X-ray evidence of severe arthritis deterioration.

Now, I grant you that this doctor wasn't used to seeing water exercise devotees who characteristically become pain-free in spite of damage to their bones and joints. But, even without knowing about water exercise there was still no sound medical basis for estimating my pain from looking at my X-rays. The fact is that while damage to bones and joints is involved in arthritis, this damage is not the direct cause of arthritis pain. And the strange thing was that the doctor knew the correct facts. When I questioned him, his answers showed that he was intellectually aware of what caused arthritis pain. Yet, his previous remarks and reactions had shown that he wasn't functionally aware.

Another event was a social conversation that I had with a recent medical-school graduate. In passing, I mentioned something about the arthritis pain-relieving benefits of water exercise. This young gentlemen reacted by looking at me incredulously. And then, as if he was trying to be polite in the face of stupidity, he answered, 'Yes but what about the bones?' Well, I gave him a few sentences of explanation and then he said something to the effect of, 'Hey, wait a minute, that's right. We learned in school that the pain in rheumatoid arthritis is caused by muscle spasms.' Again, he knew the cause of pain, yet he didn't know it. (Muscle spasms are painful muscle contractions. And they are mostly what I am referring to when I use the term 'tense, tight muscles'.)

Lastly, these two conversations inspired me to go to the public library and read the available books about arthritis. These were books written by doctors for laymen. And as far as what was explained about arthritis there was quite a bit about bones and joints and almost nothing about muscles. Believe it or not, I had to read through five books before I saw a single one-sentence explanation that mentioned the muscles as the actual cause of pain.

The importance of all this is that to the extent that doctors think, act and write this way, harm is caused to patients. The most obvious harm is in the misdirection of arthritis treatments away from treating the actual cause of pain. Less obvious, but none the less important, is the psychological damage done to patients. It can be very frightening to be told that X-rays show that there is something wrong with your bones. That has a certain inevitable sound to it. Thus if people believe, or are led to believe, that their pain is caused by their bones then they can get the feeling that there is really not much that can be done for them. There is a tendency to more or less give up hope for recovery.

15 Arthritis Pain and Water Exercise

So that you may aquire a better and more complete understanding of things, I will try to put an end to some of the existing confusion about bones, muscles and pain. Deterioration of bones and joints is involved in arthritis, but this deterioration is only one step in a chain of events that finally results in arthritis pain. With rheumatoid arthritis, the chain starts out with an X-factor — the unknown factor or factors that cause the onset of the disease. This X-factor causes damage to your joints. And part of the damage takes the form of irritation of nerves in the joint lining. This nerve irritation causes chemical changes to take place. These chemical changes cause your muscles to spasm. And it is those spasms in your muscles that actually cause your pain.

With osteoarthritis, again we start with an unknown X-factor. This X-factor causes damage to your bones. But here we have a slight variation, because osteoarthritic bone damage doesn't always result in pain and the pain that does result isn't always proportional to the damage. (For instance, you could have a little damage and a lot of pain or a lot of damage and a little pain.) So, for want of a better word, we'll say that chemical changes 'accompany' bone damage. These chemical changes then cause your muscles to spasm and it is these muscle spasms that actually cause your pain.

In addition to muscle spasms, arthritis pain can also be caused by muscle weakness. This muscle weakness results from disuse and from the disease itself. At any rate, when an arthritic tries to move one of his joints using weak, contracted muscles, part of the increased pain is caused by muscle weakness.

The following chart illustrates the chain of events that takes place to cause both rheumatoid and osteoarthritis pain.

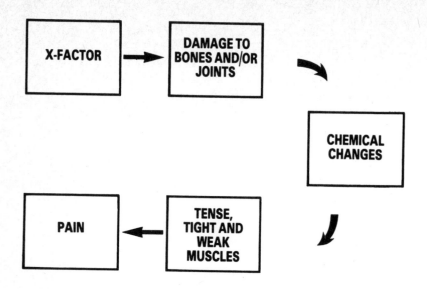

To stop your pain, what has to be done is break the chain at some point. Since no one knows what causes arthritis, it is not yet possible to treat the cause. And surgery to repair or replace bones and joints may not by itself entirely stop your pain because bone surgery does not always reverse the tendency towards muscle contractions and muscle weakness. What drug treatments try to do is alter the chemical changes that cause muscle contractions and pain. (Unfortunately, drugs also alter your body's general chemistry, thus causing the host of adverse reactions that people get from taking these drugs.)

Water exercise involves a different approach. Treatment with water exercise does not effect the cause of arthritis or reverse damage to bones and joints or stop chemical changes from taking place. Yet, water exercise really works. The way it works is by breaking the chain at its next to last point. What happens is that by gradually relaxing, stretching and strengthening your muscles, water exercise reverses the muscle spasms and muscle weakness that are actually causing your pain. Thus, by treating the actual cause of pain, you become pain-free in spite of X-ray observable damage to your bones and joints.

A diagram of the condition of a successful water exercise adherent would look like the following:

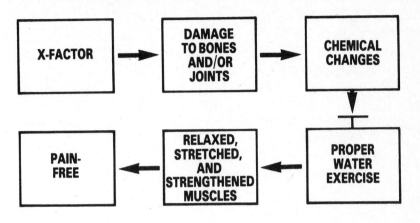

16 Limited Range of Motion and Water Exercise

Most arthritics who have a limited range of motion have seen or been told about their X-rays which show damage to their bones and joints. Thus, many arthritics tend to assume that joint damage is the sole cause of their inability to move freely. Most often these assumptions are wrong because there are two factors, not just one, that affect range of motion. These two factors are 'the condition of your joints' and 'the condition of your muscles and ligaments'. (Ligaments connect bones to one another and the same exercises that

117

benefit your muscles simultaneously benefit your ligaments.)

Of the two factors, it is much more common for the muscles (and ligaments) to be the limiting factor. Your muscles are connected to your bones (by means of tendons) and it is the movement of your muscles that makes your movement possible. In the last chapter you read how damage to bones and joints results in muscle contractions and muscle weakness. Obviously, these muscular problems contribute to making movement painful and difficult. But the answer to the question of whether water exercise can restore full range of motion depends on whether movement is actually being prevented by the joints or the muscles or both. And it depends on the particular type of joint damage involved.

One extreme type of joint damage takes the form of total bone fusion. Once bones have become totally fused together they will not move regardless of the condition of your muscles. In this case, the important limiting factor is the bones, not the muscles, and thus water exercise can be of no value. (While water exercise cannot reverse total bone fusion it can prevent it. In addition to making movement possible, muscles and ligaments act to support the skeletal system. It is the weakness and deterioration of muscles and ligaments that allows joints to collapse to the point where bone fusion becomes possible. Water exercise prevents this type of total collapse by strengthening muscles and ligaments.)

There is a second type of situation where there are two factors that are abnormally limiting the range of motion. One factor would be joint damage that takes the form of partial bone fusion (as differentiated from total bone fusion) or an extremely narrowed joint space (as differentiated from the 'normally' narrow joint space that most arthritics have). And the other limiting factor would be the weak, contracted and painful muscles that accompany these conditions. In this case, movement could be partially improved to the extent that the cause of disability is muscular. And the way to find out how much it can be improved is to go to a pool and give water exercise a chance to help. (As with total bone fusion, partial bone fusion and extremely narrow joint spaces can be prevented if water exercise is started in time.)

The third type of situation, that I'm going to describe now, is the situation that the great majority of arthritics are in. They have terrible-looking X-rays that show narrow joint spaces, bone spurs and all sorts of other abnormalities. But their bones haven't fused together and their joint spaces haven't narrowed so much that they actually prevent movement. In these cases there is only one factor that is causing a limited range of motion. Muscles are the culprits and this muscular factor can be completely reversed by water exercise.

What proper water exercise does is gradually relax, stretch and strengthen your tense, tight and weak muscles, as well as move your joints. As your muscles gradually relax, stretch and strengthen, your pain gradually decreases and your range of motion gradually increases. Eventually, you become pain-free and fully able to move in spite of X-rays' observable damage to your bones and joints.

17 Arthritis Deformities and Water Exercise

I have already explained that damage to bones and joints results in chemical changes that cause muscle contractions. What happens in many cases of arthritis deformity is that these contractions of muscles and tendons become so severe that they cause visual deformities such as crooked fingers and arthritic lumps and nodes. The way this happens is that the muscles and tendons that are connected to your bones contract so much that they move your bones out of their proper alignment. Also, tendons contract so much that they ball up into knots and thus appear as lumps or nodes.

Not all visual deformities are caused this way, but many are. The good news is that to the extent that deformities are caused by contractions of muscles and tendons they can be reversed by proper water exercise. For instance, water exercise is the reason that my once-crippled fingers now appear to be straight. X-rays might still show them to have arthritis damage, but they look straight because my muscles are no longer pulling them out of place. Similarly, nodes that I once had on my fingers are also gone.

Remember, I said that not all deformities are caused this way. So, keep in mind that while many deformities can be partially or fully reversed by water exercise, not all can. Be aware of the possibility of reversal, but don't set your hopes up too high just from reading this. If possible, find out what is causing any deformities that you may have. Also, and more importantly, see how your body reacts to proper water exercise. Until you do that you won't really know anything. All I can tell you now is that the chances for partial and full reversals of deformities are a lot greater than most doctors think they are.

In conclusion, medical science has long understood the muscular component in arthritis pain and deformity. Yet, the intellectual understanding that doctors have of this has not translated itself into effective action. The main thrust of their treatment has been drugs and surgery. Physiotherapy has been relegated to the status of a criminally painful (as with land exercise) and the ridiculously inept (as with existing water exercise programmes) throwin. It is my hope in writing this that once you become aware of the same facts that the doctors are, you will use these facts to come to different conclusions. Hopefully, you will realise the necessity for alternative action.

18 Surgery?

Responsible doctors consider surgery, in non-emergency situations, to be 'the treatment of last resort'. What that means is that before they suggest surgery, they first try to exhaust the other possibilities. They try other methods of treatment in the hope that surgery can be avoided. There is a very good reason for this. And that reason is that any surgery, even relatively 'safe' surgery, involves risks to the life and health of the patient being operated on.

There could be a bad reaction to the anaesthesia. Infection could set in. Any number of things could happen. I am not saying that they will happen, but they could happen. Death can result from even the 'safest' of operations. And that is why you should approach non-emergency surgery with even more caution than your doctor. After all, the death in question would be yours, not his.

Before agreeing to undergo any operation you should gather enough information to enable you to weigh the possible risks against the possible rewards accurately. Do not be satisfied with your doctor's statement that an operation is safe. Ask him to define 'safe' in terms of the percentage of people who have died or developed serious complications from previous operations of the type in question. Also, try to make sure that the percentage is valid for the specific hospital where the operation is supposed to take place. Survival rates, for a particular operation, can vary according to the quality of post-operative care given in different hospitals.

As far as rewards go, ask your doctor to explain in detail exactly what you can reasonably expect if the operation goes according to plan. Also, ask if you could be put in touch with some former patients who have had successful operations. Find out, from the patient's point of view, exactly how successful these operations really are.

The aforementioned suggestions represent good advice about surgery for any non-emergency condition. When it comes to arthritis I can offer you even better advice. 'Before you seriously contemplate an operation, try water exercise first. You have nothing to lose and everything to gain.'

If you ever have reason to discuss my advice with a surgeon, I suggest that you keep the following thoughts in mind:

(1) **Water exercise is not dangerous but surgery could be.**
(2) **Arthritis operations are not emergencies. Thus, temporarily delaying an arthritis operation will not cause harm.**
(3) **There are marginal cases where no one could intelligently predict beforehand how much good water exercise would do.**
(4) **Most doctors ignore the muscles and tend to think of the problem exclusively in terms of X-ray observable bone damage.**
(5) **Most doctors are aware of the limitations of standard physiotherapy and water exercise programmes, but very few are aware of how much good a good water exercise programme can do.**

I have no doubt that if the great majority of arthritics started water exercise soon enough, then the great majority of arthritis surgery could be avoided. That is a general statement. Unfortunately I can't give you specific answers about any surgery that you may be contemplating. All I can do is repeat my suggestion that you 'try water exercise first'.

If, by some chance, you should try water exercise and find that it can't help you (remember that it takes at least a couple of months to note major improvement) keep in mind that that doesn't necessarily mean that you should agree to being operated on. It doesn't necessarily follow that an effective operation exists just because you have a condition that might require an operation. As I mentioned at the beginning of this chapter, 'Before agreeing to any operation, you should gather enough information to enable you to weigh the possible risks against the possible rewards accurately.'

Also, if you do have surgery, please note the importance of following up on an operation with proper water exercise. The reason that you can have a 'successful' joint replacement without the elimination of your pain is that the joint replacement doesn't do very much for your muscles.

19 The Way Things Should Be Done

What I've been discussing so far has been reversing the pain and disability of long-term arthritis sufferers. As I have mentioned, proper water exercise does this amazingly well. But water exercise has even more value. What it can do is prevent long-term suffering from ever taking place.

Osteoarthritis is by far the most common form of arthritis. (Of the thirty-one million arthritis sufferers in the United States, sixteen million suffer from osteoarthritis, six million from rheumatoid arthritis, and the rest suffer from the ninety-plus other less-common varieties of arthritis that exist. In the United Kingdom there are six million arthritis sufferers. With serious osteoarthritis, the pain usually starts as slight pain and gradually gets worse and worse over a period of years. As the pain worsens, the standard medical treatment is to prescribe drugs. And if less powerful drugs don't control the pain, then ever more powerful drugs are prescribed.

This method of treatment is, of course, ridiculous. People should not take drugs for five, ten, or twenty years while their pain gets worse and worse. People should not have to suffer for five, ten or twenty years before they start water exercise. Water exercise should be started immediately after osteoarthritis is diagnosed. The effect of this would be to prevent the pain from ever getting worse, prevent possible joint collapse of the type that can lead to surgery, and quickly and easily eliminate the pain that does exist (the less pain you start with, the fewer months it should take you to eliminate your pain).

While there is no question that water exercise should be started immediately after osteoarthritis is diagnosed, such immediacy does not necessarily hold true for rheumatoid arthritis. With rheumatoid arthritis, there are wide variations in the characteristics and severity of the disease. One of those variations, that some people experience, is a beginning stage of the disease that involves joint inflammation that may be so severe that it may make exercise (even water exercise) imprudent. (You can exercise a joint that is very painful as long as the exercise doesn't cause increased pain. But I caution you never to exercise a joint that looks red and feels hot until the redness and heat have disappeared. I also caution you that if you have rheumatoid arthritis the best thing to do is check with your doctor before starting an exercise programme.) At any rate, once this particular beginning stage has passed or if it doesn't occur, then water exercise can be just as beneficial for rheumatoid arthritis as it is for osteoarthritis.

After the beginning stages have passed, what the patient is left with is joint damage and pain caused by the muscles. Again, the standard treatment for this employs drugs and more drugs. And again, to eliminate the pain and prevent further collapse of the joint, the much-better treatment is proper water exercise.

I know people who, as a result of water exercise, have become pain-free without any help from doctors. But that is neither the ideal nor prudent way to do things. The best way to benefit from water exercise is in co-operation with a doctor. Assuming doctors recognise the importance of water exercise, I see the medical role as the following:

(1) **Diagnosing the cause of pain. Chronic pain can be caused by other things than arthritis. Thus, it is**

important to know what you are dealing with.

(2) If the type of arthritis diagnosed is rheumatoid arthritis, doctors should tell patients when they can start their exercise programmes.

(3) Doctors should explain the benefits of water exercise and encourage their patients to try it.

(4) Patients that aren't ambulatory should be started out on water exercise in a hospital setting if this is practical.

In addition to medical co-operation, what would also be beneficial is a government-sponsored public information campaign (the drug companies certainly aren't going to spend money to publicise water exercise). The role of this campaign would be twofold. First, to inform the public that something new has been developed that can actually help them. It is necessary to inform arthritics publicly because many of them have given up on their doctor's ability to help. Consequently, there are many arthritics in need of help who are not in touch with doctors.

The second facet of this public information campaign would be to explain water exercise properly. People must not be confused into thinking that all that has been advocated is that 'arthritics should go swimming'. People must be made to understand that to achieve the kind of results that I have been talking about, they must 'do the proper exercises and follow the proper principles of exercise.' In addition to a public information campaign it would be doubly beneficial if the government made more pools available to arthritics throughout the country (and this includes Britain).

What is described above is the ideal way in which arthritis should be treated. Doing things this way involves co-operation between patients, doctors and government. I do not know whether this type of co-operation is possible. But what I do know is that treatment of this type would result in many benefits to society. In human terms, there would be much less suffering. Most new arthritics could avoid the major consequences of the disease. And most long-term sufferers could reverse their pain and disability and rejoin the mainstream of society as productive members.

In financial terms, the amount of money alternative treatment could save is almost beyond comprehension. It has been estimated that over five billion dollars a year is currently being spent on arthritis care in the United States alone. Billions more are spent world-wide. Water exercise is much less costly than surgical appliances, drugs, hospitalisation and surgery. There is no doubt that society would benefit greatly if the billions of dollars that could be saved were spent on better things.

By all means, researchers should continue to look for a safe drug that will either prevent, cure or effectively control arthritis. But until such a drug is found, emphasis must be moved away from drug treatments. Both patients and doctors must fully recognise the cause of most arthritis pain and disability. And they must make every effort to treat that cause intelligently. What is required is proper procedure and perseverance. With that, pain-free arthritis is achievable for the great majority of arthritics.

Conclusion

Most of Part Two has consisted of an overview of arthritis treatment. I have spoken in general terms about what 'is' and what 'should be'. I am going to conclude by speaking to you as an individual.

Because water exercise is not profitable for either doctors or drug companies, it is doubtful that it will ever become the standard treatment for arthritis in the US. In other parts of the world where profit isn't the major motive in medicine, water exercise may, one day, become the accepted treatment for arthritis. But change takes time. And as an individual you can't afford to wait for 'one day' to come. As an individual, you owe it to yourself to do as much for yourself as you can, as soon as you can.

I have developed the method by which you can help yourself. And the closer you follow that method, the better chance you will have of helping yourself. But, having explained water exercises to you, I have done all that I can do for you. *As an individual, it is now up to you to go out and do for yourself.*

Afterword

More on chronic back and neck pain not involving arthritis

Most arthritics and most sufferers from chronic back and neck pain not involving arthritis have three things in common with each other. The first thing is the generally ineffective medical treatment that they receive. The second thing is the similar cause of their pain. And the third thing is the great probability that they can be helped by the Berson Program. Yes, the very same program that works for arthritis also works for most chronic back and neck pain not involving arthritis.

To understand why the Berson Program works for both conditions you have to understand what causes most chronic back and neck pain. Most chronic back and neck pain involves problems with disks. What happens is that a disk becomes slightly out of place. This leads to a narrowing of the free space around a spinal nerve. (When a lot of narrowing takes place this is known as having a "pinched nerve"). When narrowing is accompanied by nerve irritation then chemical changes take place that cause muscle spasms. As with arthritis, it is these muscle spasms that are the immediate cause of pain. And as with arthritis, by gradually relaxing, stretching and strengthening your muscles you can gradually stop the pain.

In addition to treating the immediate cause of your pain the Berson Program also provides important long term benefits for your back and neck. For instance, strengthening your muscles enables them to provide better support for your skeletal system. And better support lessens the strain on your disks. Also, the movement involved in following the program helps to improve the nutrition that your disks receive. (Mature disks do not have a capillary system to bring nutrients into the disk itself. Instead, they receive their nutrition by a form of liquid absorbtion that is aided by movement.) To summarize, as a result of relaxing, stretching and strengthening your muscles, providing better support for your skeletal system, lessening the strain on your disks and improving disk nutrition, the Berson Program not only stops your pain but also makes it very unlikely that pain will reoccur. (Remember though that to prevent periodic reoccurrence you must continue with the program for the rest of your life.)

As I see it, the main medical role in treating most chronic back and neck pain should be one of providing proper diagnosis. Proper diagnosis is particularly important because in approximately 2% of cases chronic pain could be caused by tumors, infections, or rare bone diseases that require forms of treatment that are very different from what I'm discussing. (If the cause of your pain has already been correctly diagnosed then you shouldn't worry. If you have chronic pain that hasn't yet been diagnosed you shouldn't worry either but you should have the cause of your pain determined as accurately as possible.)

Another thing that your doctor can tell you that I can also tell you is to use common sense about when to start your exercise program. If you are having an acute attack of pain that makes it almost impossible to get out of bed then obviously you shouldn't try to drag yourself to a pool until this acute stage has passed. And needless to say, when you get to a pool you should follow the same guidelines as the people with arthritis about not straining yourself.

The reason I think the formal medical role should be limited mostly to diagnosis is that I don't think very much of the current medical treatments.

Specifically:

1) Traction of the type I did for my neck is not only painful but it also has very little history of effectiveness.

2) Collars and corsets may provide temporary relief but they do not provide any sort of long term solution. In fact, it is possible to argue

that the immobility involved in wearing them on a long term basis has a negative effect on disk nutrition, circulation and muscle strength. (Regardless of the above, if you are currently dependent on a collar or a corset you should not immediately stop using it. What you should do is gradually use it less and less as you gradually get better from the Berson Program.)

3) Heat treatments, such as whirlpool treatments, may provide some temporary relief but they do not provide progressive improvement of the type that leads to major long term benefits. Whatever relief you get from heat treatments results from the fact that heat causes your muscles to temporarily relax and stretch. The reason heat treatments don't result in major dramatic improvement is because they don't relax and stretch your muscles nearly as much as proper water exercise does. And the reason heat brings only temporary relief is because your muscles rapidly contract back to their original state of tightness soon after they are removed from the source of the heat.

4) The Berson Program can make most operations for chronic back and neck pain unnecessary. But aside from that, even if the Berson Program didn't exist, you should be aware that this type of surgery is expensive, involves some risk and has a generally poor history of success. "Before submitting to any operation for chronic back and neck pain you should investigate thoroughly both your specific need for an operation and the operation's specific history of success". (For a more complete discussion of surgery read the chapter on arthritis surgery.)

5) Many doctors recognize the theoretical benefits of exercise for chronic back and neck pain. Thus many doctors recommend exercise to their patients. A major problem with most of the exercise that they recommend is the same problem that exists with the arthritis exercise that most doctors recommend. And that is that it is almost impossibly painful for someone who is already in pain to exercise on land. Additionally, some of the exercise programs recommended by doctors are difficult to do even for people not in pain. And finally, none of these land programs incorporate all of the best movements for your back and neck.

6) Some doctors do suggest to their patients that they try swimming for back and neck pain. And some even suggest that their patients do the backstroke. While this advice points patients in the right general direction it is far from specific enough. In fact, it is almost comparable to telling a patient,"Go to the drug store and buy some sort of drug and then swallow it when you feel like it". While some people may improve

from this type of advice it is only because they happen to accidentally do the right thinngs in the water. Of course, if you want less dependence on chance and much greater probability of becoming pain-free, then instead of just "going swimming" you should follow the Berson Program.

Because of the increased twisting and stretching it involves, the Berson version of the back stroke is much better for your back than the Olympic version. But it still won't do everything for your back. " For the greatest certainty of improvement, you should do all the exercises in this book that apply to your area of pain, you should do the exercises in a mechanically correct manner and you should follow the proper principles of exercise ". (An example of a good comprehensive program for your back would be to eventually work up to doing a combination of exercises 21, 31, 34, and 35.)

It is interesting to note that doctors have long been aware of anecdotal evidence that some patients with arthritis and/or chronic back pain got a lot of benefit from swimming. It is also interesting to note that at the same time doctors have also been aware that many patients received little or no benefit from swimming. What is most interesting is that the medical conclusion from this was that water exercise could be of some benefit to some people but it was very far from being the major answer for the problems of arthritis and chronic back and neck pain. Of course, the fallacy of this conclusion is that it is based on the false assumptions that 1) all water exercise is the same 2) all exercise done in water is equally correct and helpful. Apparently, no one bothered to consider that the people who benefitted most from water exercise did so primarily because they happened to be exercising in a more correct manner (in terms of type, amount and frequency of exercise) than the people that benefitted least. Apparently, no one prior to myself realized that the degree of correctness was the major factor in determining the degree of benefit. Thus, I was the first to realize that if everyone exercised in a perfectly correct manner then almost everyone would benefit to some degree and most people would become totally pain-free.

In conclusion, if you suffer from the type of chronic back and neck pain that most people suffer from then you are probably suffering needlessly. My advice to you is to try the program, follow it correctly and find out for yourself how much you can be helped.